D0000344

The Gut Solution

FOR PARENTS WITH CHILDREN WHO HAVE
RECURRENT ABDOMINAL PAIN
AND IRRITABLE BOWEL SYNDROME

By
Michael Lawson, MD, and Jessica Del Pozo, PhD

Illustrations: Ryan Walter

Design and Production: Amy Bishop

ISBN-13: 978-0615879758
ISBN-10: 0615879756

DEDICATION

This book is dedicated with love to our supportive and patient spouses, Helen and Carlos.

Acknowledgments

We sing highest praises to Monica and Bob Randel and Andre Shaw for the energy and creativity that they have brought to the treatment of children with IBS for many years; as well as Tashia Orr for her hard work, flexibility, and persistence enrolling families into the IBS program.

Nancy Gronert is the teacher we are ever grateful to who triggered a "light-bulb moment" for Mike about the severity of functional digestive problems in middle-school-age children.

Rhonda Gage RN, Michael Durant MD and Pratime Kodali MD contributed their time and energy to the program.

We also sincerely thank Jeremy Katz for his way with words and getting the book off the ground at the very beginning. We wish him the best on his future writing endeavors.

We thank our incredibly valuable readers for lending many hours of personal and professional expertise to improve the rough manuscript toward a finished product: Jackie Brown, Matt Kurowski, Jeffrey Lemke, Carlos Del Pozo, Emily, Peter and Elyse Lawson, and Carol Davies.

We thank the talented data crunchers who have shown us scientifically that our program is effective: Andrea Griem, Leslie Crebassa, and Amir Kalani.

We appreciate our many friends who have allowed us to talk about gastrointestinal topics (frequently over dinner) and shared their stories with us, as well as the many dear people who have encouraged us to keep writing despite our busy schedules.

And last, but certainly not least, thank you to all of the families, children and parents who participated in the IBS program, as well as our families for all of your love and support.

Many sincere thanks,

Mike and Jessica

Disclaimer

This book is not meant to take the place of direct medical diagnosis and treatment.

You must not rely on the information in this book as an alternative to medical advice from your doctor or other professional healthcare provider. If you have specific questions about any medical matter you should consult your doctor or other professional healthcare providers.

If you think your child may be suffering from any organic medical condition you should seek immediate medical attention. You should never delay seeking medical advice, disregard medical advice, or discontinue medical treatment because of information in this book.

Contents

PART II: PLANTING THE SEEDS

Introduction

A Word By Dr. Lawson

This book arose from my determination to reduce unnecessary suffering in my adult patients with IBS. I was always impressed with the effectiveness of education and reassurance in helping patients gain insight into their problems. The end result is an improvement in symptoms by relieving the stress of the unknown. I started a successful adult IBS group-appointment program eighteen years ago. Only one in five adults attending that program requested further specialist consultation and investigation. However, I knew there was more I could do for people with IBS.

I'm a pragmatic sort, an Aussie doc who put myself through medical school by driving a cab. I have a practical practitioner's bent to me, born of the pioneer spirit that still emanates from my homeland, and it frustrates me to see patients suffer year after year, when there is a solution.

I didn't know my way around Sydney when I got my taxi license, but I sorted it out before long. The same goes for this gastrointestinal disorder—I didn't know how to solve this problem, but I knew it could be solved and I knew it was crucial that I do so.

Irritable bowel syndrome is a lesser known, yet highly prevalent and incredibly problematic chronic syndrome in the United States. IBS, as it is called, affects fully 20 percent of the population. That is sixty million people in America alone, and our health care system forks over thirty billion dollars to promote inadequate treatment and unnecessary procedures. As a gastroenterologist with several decades of clinical experience treating IBS, thirty-four research studies, and sixty publications under my belt, I can tell you that the vast majority of those dollars are wasted.

IBS won't show up on a single test, it won't respond well to drugs, and it won't simply go away with time. IBS is associated with multiple comorbidities (other diagnoses that people often have at the same time) that are among the most common complaints people have: chronic headaches, back pain, temporomandibular joint problems, chronic fatigue, depression, and anxiety. Adult sufferers of IBS—80 percent of them women—get so habituated to the condition that it becomes part of their identity. "Hi," you can hear them saying by way of introduction, "my name is Jennifer, and I am a sales manager and I have IBS." Once an adult IBS patient walks into my office, something that happens upward of six times every single day, it seems too late. The pattern is so deeply ingrained that the most effective approach struggles to take root in an adult mind that has already overly identified itself with this disorder.

When a friend and middle-school teacher asked me why so many of her students—especially girls—missed school for doctor appointments, I felt like I emerged from a time tunnel. I knew how children exhibiting early signs of IBS were going to be as adults: people living a fairly debilitated life. I wanted to help and try to stop IBS when it first showed up. I had to help these people before it became part of their identity—before they became adults. I had to solve this problem before it became deeply entrenched.

IBS and functional dyspepsia are just as severe among children. Some studies estimate that 30 percent of school-age children have IBS and RAP (recurrent abdominal pain), but I would put the number somewhat lower, between 15 percent and 20 percent. That's still a heck of a lot of children, and while many of them won't become terribly debilitated like the people I see every day, I can guarantee that every single one of them suffers, and suffers needlessly.

About seven years ago, I created the SEEDS program. Working with a team of skilled practitioners, I designed a five-part protocol that treats IBS with no drugs and no major restrictions. I was fortunate to have Dr. Del Pozo join soon after, completing the picture for the comprehensive mind and body intervention we offer.

Over four hundred adolescents have attended with great success. If you have IBS, you may be dealing with it for the rest of your life, but with the SEEDS program, children with IBS learn to make this disorder a barely noticeable part of a healthy, successful life.

A Word By Dr. Del Pozo

I grew up the daughter of a football coach. "No pain, no gain" was part of life. "Life is hard, get a helmet" was not unheard of in my Midwestern upbringing. And indeed, life is hard for everyone at times. I finished college with degrees in psychology and art, foolishly thinking that my table-waiting days were over. I quickly realized I was now a more interesting waitress with a ton of debt, and decided to continue my education to learn about things that interested me.

My curiosity about the mind-body connection grew partially from my own experience in sports. I pitched for women's fast pitch softball, ran track, played broomball and rugby, and was always ready for a pickup football game (and still am). To have the edge as an athlete, it seemed that one needed to have "one's head in the game." Physical fitness and discipline certainly mattered, coaching was key, but without a clear and focused mind, performance was still hindered. What people believed about themselves seemed to make the good athletes great and the great ones good. Beliefs could also make the great ones choke.

I noticed the same held true for health. I have worked with medical populations for over fifteen years, academically in research settings as well as clinically. Each year that goes by, each talk, each patient, I learn something new. I understand more and more how intricately the mind and body work together. The impact of stress is more recognized now than ever by the medical community, but the message is falling short on its journey to the patient. Many patients hear "it's just stress" and are left worried that something else is wrong or, at best, wondering what to do about it. Chronic stress makes us ill. When we believe we are helpless or trapped in our lives, when we feel alone, it directly impacts our health and quality of life through a number of pathways. Chronic back pain, headaches, digestive complaints, disrupted sleep, and fatigue are common complaints no matter what setting I have worked in. I want people to understand themselves better and to feel more in control of their symptoms, which means feeling more in control of their lives.

I joined Dr. Lawson shortly after he had gathered together our team of movement, relaxation, and diet experts to help children with IBS and

RAP. I am continually impressed with his understanding of the intricacies of the oh-so complicated gastrointestinal tract, as well as his ability to see the forest *and* the trees within what has become a somewhat stigmatized problem.

While there are many important factors to consider in managing a life with IBS, the five prongs of SEEDS encompass the bio-psycho-social model of medicine rather than a strictly biological or psychological one. By fully understanding each of the components listed below from biological and psychological perspectives within a social context—and how they are connected to digestive health—SEEDS can free you and your children from the potential traps of IBS.

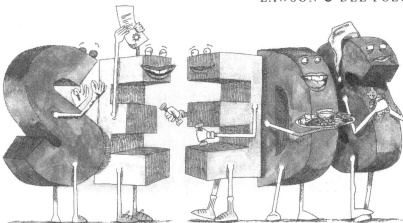

STRESS MANAGEMENT

This includes intentional and regular relaxation, thinking about what is stressful in a new way, not buying into your thoughts all the time, challenging your beliefs, accepting feelings for what they are, and seeking help for anxiety and depression when necessary.

EDUCATION AND REASSURANCE

This includes learning facts about IBS, dispelling myths, and accepting reassurance that IBS is real, but not life threatening. It is about learning how to communicate better and more assertively; setting healthy, consistent, loving, and supportive limits; and, most of all, listening to each other.

EXERCISE

Daily movement is a necessary good for the body and mind and gut. It is best in moderation, practiced frequently, and incorporated with something enjoyable. There are four main reasons to exercise for IBS, four types of exercises, and four examples of each.

DIET

Diet includes what and especially how you eat for IBS symptoms. Diet can be altered to manage diarrhea, constipation, gas, and bloating, as well as stomach pain. Do not be rigid or controlling with food, but nurture an enjoyable relationship with your child and food. Trust your child will eat what he or she needs from the good options you prepare.

SLEEP

Schedule enough time for sleep and keep a regular sleep-wake routine that includes waking the same time every day. Avoid sleeping in and do not spend time in bed worrying. There are many internal and external influences on sleep, and it is something we can train our brains to do better.

Planning for Sowing the Seeds: Socializing and Success

Feeling connected to others is another key component to a healthy life, and it helps reduce pain and suffering. Reach out to others rather than isolating when IBS symptoms flare up. Making gradual, realistic changes will likely lead to more long-lasting success over time. Integrating fun into each activity (eating, exercise, relaxation, work) will make everything easier.

Almost four in ten Americans suffer from a functional gastrointestinal disorder, but there is relief. We are committed to providing the best possible solution to you and your family for IBS, and we hope you remain committed to doing your best to apply this knowledge to your daily lives.

(Please note that he and she are used interchangeably for readability.)

> **?** Throughout this book, look out for the **'Questions for Your Family'** section at the end of each chapter to help you discuss these issues with your children.

The Language

Irritable bowel syndrome, recurrent abdominal pain, functional dyspepsia, and acid reflux disease are all functional gastrointestinal disorders (FGIDs). For the purposes of this book, we most often speak of IBS, but in doing so, we usually mean any of the functional gastrointestinal disorders. See the definitions below.

Functional gastrointestinal disorder (FGIDs): chronic or recurrent gastrointestinal discomfort, pain, or other symptoms that do not have an identified underlying disease pathology, but are marked by troublesome symptoms within the digestive tract.

Irritable bowel syndrome (IBS): symptoms related to bowel movements (diarrhea, constipation, or alternating), a sense of incomplete rectal evacuation, mucus with stool, or abdominal bloating or distention (the most common of the FGIDs).

Recurrent or functional abdominal pain (RAP): stomach pain three times per month or more that lacks an organic cause (no biochemical or physiological disease process).

Functional dyspepsia: feeling full with small amounts of food; nausea, vomiting, burping, or bloating.

PART I

Understanding the Problem

CHAPTER 1

An Overview

A Brief History of IBS and How SEEDS Can Help

Irritable bowel syndrome was first recognized as a medical problem nearly two hundred years ago, originally called an "attack of the va-pors." Today, it is the number one reason that people are referred to see a gastroenterologist. Over half of the patients these doctors see daily have IBS.

> **Chyme:**
>
> The semifluid of enzymes and partially digested food that moves from the stomach and small intestine to the large intestine.

For many years, medical care providers blamed IBS symptoms on abnormal intestinal motility—the ability of the guts to move the in-

> **Intestinal Motility:**
>
> The ability of the digestive tract to rhythmically move food along by squeezing and relaxing.

testinal chyme spontaneously while consuming energy. Doctors assumed that the pain came from an intestinal spasm, and so they named it "spastic colon" or "spastic bowel syndrome." Over time, research linked stress to the disorder, and now psychological disorders such as anxiety and depression are frequently seen along with IBS—over 60 percent of the time. As you may know, however, this does not make the physical problem of IBS any less real.

There is such a strong interconnection between stress and gut responses that emotional stress can trigger bowel hypermotility (an overactive response, such as diarrhea) in people both with and without IBS.

An early experiment found stress caused spasms and engorgement of the blood vessels in the intestinal mucosa (lining) during a sigmoidoscopy (a scope of part of the colon) when unsuspecting medical students were told by investigators, "You have cancer." Just think back to that first big presentation you gave—how did your breakfast go down that day?

IBS is diagnosed if the symptoms of pain, diarrhea, constipation, and gas or bloating become frequent and chronic. Food increases the motion of the colon fifteen minutes after the start of a meal, accounting for some of the symptoms people have after eating. However, changes in the gut's motility generally do not correlate with IBS symptoms, and medications that slow down gut motility have not been very effective. A better understanding of IBS arose through knowledge of "central" mechanisms—the central nervous system's connection to digestion. Errors in central processing of signals (to the brain and spinal cord) from the gut are of primary importance in the vast majority of people with IBS. This means that people with IBS have brains that interpret normal digestion as a painful experience, and the gut responds to the brain's interpretations by sending out a flurry of gut responses.

Studies of metabolic and biochemical activity in the brain show that people with IBS have increased activity in the prefrontal cortex—an area associated with anxiety and hypervigilence (an elevated level of sensory sensitivity and behavioral response). These people were also found to have reduced activity in the anterior cingulated cortex—an area for endorphin binding in the brain. Stress, anxiety, and depression change in accordance with sensory processing and can increase the perception of pain. Treatments that focus on only the digestive tract may not be nearly as successful as a multisystem approach that treats both the GI tract and the central nervous system. It's interesting that 85 percent of adults diagnosed with fibromyalgia also have IBS. The same is true for chronic fatigue syndrome, as well as chronic pelvic pain; half of people diagnosed with one have the other. Sixty-four percent of people with temporomandibular joint pain also have IBS. Studying these chronic health problems continues to lead us toward understanding IBS as a central nervous system disregulation.

Syndromes Connected with IBS

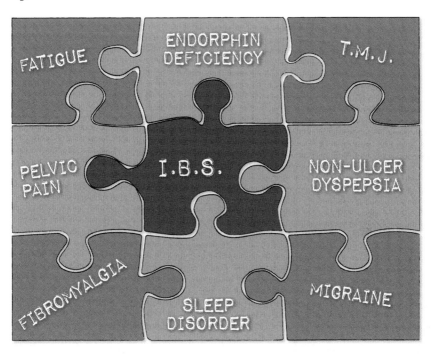

There is more. The number of CT scans done on children in the emergency room has skyrocketed in the past decade without improving doctors' ability to diagnose intestinal problems. Tests are often done simply because they can be, and sometimes done indiscriminately at the patient's insistence. More tests lead to more surgeries. Adults with IBS are 87 percent more likely to have abdominal and pelvic surgeries. They are three times as likely to have their gall bladders out and twice as likely to have hysterectomies and appendectomies. Unfortunately, removing functioning parts does not help IBS and sometimes causes more pain. This is reason enough for us to focus on preventing today's children from suffering more useless surgeries as adults. Our research and the SEEDS program have been growing over the last seven years into a multidisciplinary, evidence-based program that helps elementary-school-age children and teens with IBS.

Walking through SEEDS with Sara, a fourteen-year-old girl with IBS

When the SEEDS program was just a seedling, helping one in five children seemed a hopeful goal. Now, seven years after it began, our success rate is close to four in five children. Children who have completed SEEDS have fewer pointless x-rays and fewer needless pediatric appointments. Children with IBS generally see a gastroenterologist between ten and twelve times per year before they enter the program. After starting SEEDS, that number drops to fewer than two visits each year. And it is not just the gut symptoms that improve. Headaches disappear, sleep problems vanish, gut pain flees, and school absenteeism lessens (one of the biggest problems facing children with IBS). The benefits are durable, lasting over four years thus far in our research.

While its effects are amazing, the SEEDS program is no miracle cure. It takes work and commitment from the child and family alike, but it can make the difference between simply existing and tolerating life, and thriving and savoring it.

You may have been dragging your ailing child around to many medical appointments, trying test after test to figure out what is wrong and what to do about it. Many parents who have a child with IBS have suffered as well and shared their losses with us. They include:

- Time away from work.
- Attention away from the other children in the family.
- Lost sleep worrying about what is going on with your child.
- Loss of fun family activities due to unexpected flare-ups.

Meanwhile, your child has missed school and suffered stomachache after stomachache, unmanageable bowel movements or urgency, and mounting fears, and may have already begun to withdraw from people and activities he cares about. Often around this crisis point, pediatricians send these children to us.

This was the case with Sara, a fourteen-year-old girl with stomach cramps and revolving episodes of diarrhea and constipation. It seemed to start after she had a terrible flu a year and a half earlier with horrendous vomiting. Since then, seemingly random flares of stomach pain and diarrhea would come during school or while on vacation, which led her to think it was not related to stress. However, the churning and nausea did seem to come more often in the mornings and worsen in August, just as school began.

Sara missed several exams and soccer try-outs because of IBS. She decided against joining chorus for fear of having to excuse herself too often to find a restroom. The last family vacation to the beach was stressful as her parents and brother tried to plan around her bathroom needs. Her mother felt beside herself with worry. She had been running herself ragged making doctor appointments and even a visit to the emergency room one Sunday night. Nothing they did seemed to help. Sara's father was worried also, but frequently gone on long business trips. He felt frustrated with the chaos IBS created and confused about how worried to be. Sara's father suspected she was using it to avoid school, although she made great effort to get ready early and go. Eventually, Sara's pediatric gastroenterologist referred her to the SEEDS program. She was not particularly thrilled about going to another appointment for her digestive problems. She felt embarrassed, but desperate for help.

Sara, along with her parents and several other families, walked into the SEEDS classroom on the first floor of our medical office building where Monica, a registered dietician, greeted them with healthy snacks, samples of nondairy milks, and some high-fiber foods. Monica wrote each team member's name on the dry-erase board, explaining the role of each specialist:

- An adult gastroenterologist (or gut specialist)
- A registered dietician
- A physical trainer
- A behavioral health educator
- A clinical health psychologist
- A pediatric gastroenterologist

Each member of this multidisciplinary team would contribute to each family's understanding of IBS. Monica said, "I know it seems like food is the cause of IBS, but it isn't!" This surprised Sara and her mom. Monica explained more about food's role in IBS, including what foods can make IBS flare-ups worse (such as sugary and fatty foods, as well as eating too fast), and the various foods that can help bloating, diarrhea, constipation, or gas. At this point, Sara and the other children were sent off to have some fun with Bob, a physical trainer. Bob gave each child a stability exercise ball and showed them exercises to practice at home to build core strength as well as relax their often-cramping midsections.

Back in the classroom, the parents heard Dr. Lawson — the gastrointestinal specialist and IBS expert — talk about the brain-gut connection, helping everyone understand this functional disorder better. With several plastic brains in hand, he explained the connection between our brains and digestive tracts. Dr. Lawson described the pathway that pain takes through the gut to the brain and introduced terms like *pain gate, visceral hypersensitivity*, and *accommodation* (see chapter 2).

With flushed and somewhat happier faces, the children returned from exercising to rejoin their parents for questions and answers with Dr. Lawson. Sara felt more at ease now in the class, as well as with her diagnosis of IBS.

At home that week, Sara chose vegetarian pizza over pepperoni and limited her portion to half of what she normally ate. She tried switching cow's milk out for almond milk, and started sitting on the stability ball while doing homework and going for short walks with her mom after dinner. Sara and her family set the dinner atmosphere in their home to be relaxing. Sara stopped doing her homework at the table, and her brother turned the television off and played music instead. They all helped with the changes and felt the benefits of a leisurely dinner.

For week two of SEEDS, Sara's family and the other families from the previous week met a pediatric gastroenterologist, as well as Dr. Del Pozo, a health psychologist, Monica, the nutritionist from week one, and Andre, a health educator. Each played a role in helping children and parents learn how all of the components of SEEDS matter for improving the symptoms of IBS. The pediatric gastroenterologist answered parents' questions about what is really happening inside the intestines, allayed any myths, answered medication questions, and reas-

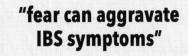

"fear can aggravate IBS symptoms"

sured parents that although very real, IBS is not dangerous or fatal.

Dr. Del Pozo spoke about the role of stress in IBS and how emotions, especially fear, can aggravate IBS symptoms. She and the families discussed parenting challenges, the importance of routine—sleeping, eating, exercising, and relaxation—as well as ways to support children with IBS while they attend school. Parents learned how they could help their children manage general anxiety as well as anxiety about IBS, in particular. Most importantly, Dr. Del Pozo discussed the importance of healthy social connections and having fun together.

The children, meanwhile, had already gone next door with Andre to put movement and relaxation skills into practice right away. They learned strenuous exercises and competed in wall squats, planks, and four-point balance. Next, Andre transitioned to stretching and yoga, concluding with relaxation techniques. He introduced the children to the importance of breathing during stretching to help oxygenate their muscles and achieve a deeper and more sustained stretch. Deep breathing also helped them understand how their conscious abilities (breathing) affect how they feel emotionally and physically.

While the children finished the last stretching exercises, Andre dimmed the lights and took them through guided imagery — a visualization practice that diminishes the intensity of unpleasant physical responses to stress. He asked them to visualize themselves in an elevator as it went down and to feel more relaxed at each level.

In this brief time, these children:

- Socialized with their peers and realized they are not alone.

- Learned what and how to eat (as well as dietary guidelines that are general and symptom-specific).

- Experienced valuable relaxation techniques and received a relaxation CD for take-home practice.

- Utilized a variety of movement skills on an exercise ball.
- Ate snack leftovers from Monica's taste test.

All the key elements of managing IBS had been introduced: social support, moving, relaxing, eating, and learning the truth about IBS.

This playful environment was packed full of knowledge for parents and offered a positive experience for children, who learned how to do simple things to help themselves cope with IBS. The shame disappeared as they realized many children (and adults) have IBS, and they felt hope for an easier future.

In three short hours, Sara and her parents were pointed in the right direction and armed with information to put it into practice right away. The comfort of having all their questions answered gave them new confidence to move forward on this journey. What they do with it could bring transitory relief or become a long-term solution for IBS.

CHAPTER SUMMARY

- Move forward from the idea that there is one cure out there for IBS, and refocus on a multifaceted approach to manage it.

- SEEDS encompasses the elements that matter: Stress management, Exercise, Education, Diet, Sleep, and Social connectedness.

- In The Gut Solution, we intend to help you apply each of these healthy behaviors to specifically manage the symptoms of IBS.

- It is very possible to have an excellent quality of life with a chronic condition like IBS.

❓ QUESTIONS FOR YOUR FAMILY

Each family member can take a turn answering the following questions.

- What things would you do if you did not have IBS? How is it different from what you do now?
- How can you begin to do those things now, with IBS?

CHAPTER 2

The Brain-Gut Axis

What Is Going on in My Gut?

The human digestive tract is staggeringly complicated. It is both compact (small enough to fit in your torso) and enormous (laid flat, the small bowel would cover a tennis court). It is part brain, part immune system, and part muscle, all linked up into a long tube that forms our most intimate connection with the outside world—the place where we literally incorporate our environment into our very bodies. The bagel and cream cheese you bought from the cart on the corner does not just magically give you energy once you gobble it down at your desk. Each bite gets ground up and mixed with salivary enzymes in your mouth before taking the elevator down to your stomach. There it gets pulverized and mixed further until there are no particles larger than four microns in size, as small as the period at the end of this sentence. This stew of ground-up food and digestive enzymes moves on to the duodenum and the small bowel, where fat, protein, and sugar—the macronutrients that make our metabolism possible—are broken down and absorbed by the body. What is left is called chyme, and it travels to the large bowel—a simple organ. All the large bowel, or colon, does is extract the water from the chyme, moving it along until it comes out as, you guessed it, poop. When this is all working well, it is a seamless process, the double-play team of digestion: breakfast to chyme to poop.

Surprisingly, for people with IBS, the basic mechanics of digestion work just fine. But how you feel during the process depends on something called accommodation, the automatic adjustment of the stomach and intestines that makes room for food. The stomach, small intestine, and colon must all accommodate the added volume of food just put into them, the chyme passing through them, and the stool accumulating—until it is time to read the paper, so to speak. There is a welter of signals that travel up the spine to your brain about your digestive state at any given moment. Messages about satiety (fullness) speed along next to information on the amount of food inside the bowels. Breakfast has its composition analyzed, its speed clocked, and its size determined. The cells that send these missives along are so much a part of the nervous system that doctors do not really think of the gut and the brain as separate organs. Instead, we speak of the brain-gut axis.

All of these messages pass up the dorsal horns of the spinal column on to a region in the midbrain called the anterior cingulate cortex. This is the body's pain gate, the tight threshold that determines if a message is alarming and if that alarm is important enough to rise to the level of consciousness. The interpretation of the pain gate, the volume control, if you will, is set up in the executive suite of the brain: the prefrontal cortex, which is responsible for higher-level, complicated processes, decisions, and social behaviors. In normal physiology, the pain gate is amplified up to a nice middle level during digestion, like easy listening—you feel it, but it's typically not bothersome. People with IBS have the volume cranked up much higher, thus feeling much more discomfort and pain than someone without IBS. This partially explains why people with IBS frequently suffer from backaches, headaches, fatigue, sleep disruption, anxiety, and depression.

To understand this better, imagine two balloons—one twice the size of the other. Give the big one a few tugs and hold it up to your lips. Several deep breaths later, it is nice and big and full. (Twisting it into an elephant is purely extra credit.) The balloon easily accommodated the volume of air you put into it. Now take the smaller balloon and repeat the process, putting exactly the same amount of air into it. It did not accommodate the same volume of air so well, did it? (Sorry about the big pop.) Similarly, as the gut of someone with IBS fills with food, liquid, and gas, it sends a crush of signals that pass through the pain gate unhampered, to be read by the prefrontal cortex as pain. The gut is supremely accommodating, like that big balloon, but the brain of a person with IBS mistakenly perceives that it is more like the small balloon—liable to pop at any moment.

A nice analogy, but what about in real life, with real balloons? In fact, when actual balloons are inserted into the large bowels of people with IBS, discomfort is felt at half the volume compared to people without IBS. In other words, people with IBS have digestive tracts twice as sensitive as people without it. We call this phenomenon visceral hypersensitivity. Pain in IBSers is often migratory and may move to other places in the body. In Germany, they jokingly call IBS the "und-here" syndrome. When people are asked to localize their pain, they point all over to different regions of the abdomen, saying, "I haf pain here, und here, und here, und here." This is because the whole GI tract can suffer from visceral hypersensitivity.

Visceral Hypersensitivity
Visceral refers to internal organs and hypersensitivity refers to information flooding the brain with sensations that are interpreted more strongly than expected.

If that were the end of the issues with accommodation, then IBS would be simple to solve. However, this digestive hypersensitivity sets up a whole cascade of problems. Let's go back to the balloons, but this time, use two balloons of the same size. Blow up the first one the normal way. Stuff the second one into a water glass. Now try to blow it up to the same size. Once again, you were thwarted. The gut of a person with IBS is like a balloon constrained by a water glass. When the pain gate lets inappropriate signals through to the prefrontal cortex, a corresponding tension reaction is sent back down those same message pathways. The prefrontal cortex floods the body with stress hormones and tells the smooth muscles of the gut to tighten up. Now the already impaired accommodation of the digestive tract is made even worse, and yet louder signals go rocketing up to that wide open pain gate. A terrible feedback loop of discomfort starts reinforcing itself, and an IBS flare is born.

Stinking pain receptors—can't we just get rid of them? We all have pain receptors throughout our bodies, and truly this is a good thing. At times you may wish you did not feel pain, but really, without feeling the sting of a bee or an achy muscle, life would be very short. (In fact, there is a disorder where people are born without pain receptors.) Without sensors telling us what feels good and what does not, our bodies would not know when to shift from one position to another, when to sweat, when our hand is touching a hot stove, or when we are hungry. We need pain receptors to tell us when to change something (like "take your hand out of that fire!").

So, some pain messages are good, but sometimes that message overplays itself and is not helpful. Chronic pain can send the brain messages that something is hurting when in fact nothing is wrong. The more the message is sent, the wider and deeper that neural (nerve or chemical) pathway becomes. Over time, it becomes more sensitive and more difficult to quiet down.

There are a withering number of additional wrinkles in this story involving gut flora balance, bowel neurotransmitter receptors, and overactive mast cells, but when it comes to how people with IBS feel, it all comes down to this wide open pain gate. The earlier that pathway is created and the longer it stays, the more challenging it is to change later in life. The good news is that because of neuroplasticity (growing new neuron pathways and altering connections), it is possible to change these messages. Many things influence the pain gate to widen and increase the noise (adverse life events, negative emotional states, inactivity, certain foods) and many things help close the gate and soften the noise (good sleep, fun activities, helping others, exercise, relaxation). We plan to teach you how to have more control over the pain gate.

Neuroplasticity

The capacity of the nervous system to regenerate or make new neuronal connections (nerve connections).

Are My Genes Too Tight?

Although IBS is four times more common in a child with a parent who has IBS, no single gene or genetic change in the sixty candidate genes has been found directly linked to IBS. This makes sense, as there is no single way that IBS manifests itself. There are numerous common nerve receptors in our intestines and brains that determine how we react to chemicals, such as serotonin, when released from our nerve endings. You might have heard of serotonin before as an important regulator of mood. As it turns out, there are many more serotonin receptors in our intestines than in our brains. Genes also determine which receptors get activated and deactivated, to what degree, and when. For Sara, our fourteen-year-old IBS patient, these receptors are on high alert when she is taking an exam at school or entering the cafeteria, but not so for her brother.

So, does this mean it is genetic, learned, environmental, or something else? The simple answer is yes, all of the above. Our environment and what we learn consciously or otherwise (subconsciously, unconsciously) is intertwined with our DNA, each affecting the other in marvelous ways. To tease out the role of each is more difficult. Studies comparing twins raised together to twins raised separately have tried to explain the role of environment versus DNA on the next generation. This is difficult, though, as the two cannot be completely isolated (remember, they shared Mom's uterus for the first nine months). However, experts in this area have estimated that roughly half of who we are is determined by our genetics. That leaves the other half of ourselves to be impacted by factors in our environment—some controllable and some not. What we choose each day to do with our bodies (exercise, relaxation, diet, socializing, hobbies, work) does make a difference. Recently, one study found that daily stress impacted health more than smoking and alcohol use together! But before you run out for a pack of cigarettes and a six-pack, the point is to try to control the things we can and not worry about the rest.

Genetics are often compared to a building blueprint. The blueprint, or plan, is laid out, but what actually comes to fruition depends on permits, various contractors, practicality, and other hurdles along the way. Bill may be hardwired with the genetic blueprint to have diabetes, but stressful events and learned daily habits (sleep, diet, exercise, stress management) can trigger the disease from potentiality into actuality. The same is true for the brain-gut connection in IBS. A perfect answer to the age-old nature-or-nurture question is unnecessary for us to move forward in pursuit of good health. Both environment and genes impact us at every level, and even a most sensitive digestive system can be improved with consistent lifestyle changes. Easier said than done, right? The good news is that we do not have to have a degree in genetic engineering to start feeling better.

Although the symptoms of IBS are exacerbated by chronic stress as well as unhealthy living habits, geneticists are finding that stress also directly affects which genes get expressed from our genetic blueprint. The digestive tract is especially sensitive, as it is directly connected to the brain's emotional and mood-processing centers. These centers reside in our brains near the control centers for pain and sleep. Often the gut is responding to stress before we even realize what is happening. It is, in fact, quite common for people with digestive disorders to also have headaches and body pain (jaw, back, chest) and trouble sleeping. Pain is often the physical manifestation of stress. After all, all that tension must reside somewhere. It is not just in our heads.

With a wide open pain gate and entrenched neurological signals, along with a genetic propensity for a sensitive gut, children with IBS feel every little sensation. And their brains interpret these signals as horrible. Add a little stress to that, and boom, a disheartening, debilitating flare-up. Our sensitivity to pain varies as much as our sensitivities to stress. Our genetics may determine the degree of our particular stress response, but what is perceived as stressful also varies from person to person. One of your children may simply have a lower threshold for pain or nausea than another. Or perhaps your child with IBS has a lower threshold for fear than your other children. Together, their experiences are quite different. Let's take an example.

Sara's older brother, Josh, has always been excited about school and navigated his academic and social worlds quite well. Sara is less extroverted and is intimidated by homework and by her peers. Josh naturally looks forward to each day and thrives being involved in baseball and the speech club. The last thing Sara wants is to speak in front of people, and she feels incredibly anxious before tests. She gets diarrhea and uses the bathroom frequently during class and fears being teased by her classmates if they notice how long she is gone. Staying focused during exams is difficult as she fears she will need the bathroom. A slight dip in test scores increases her anxiety about returning to school each day. Over time, just thinking about school triggers her stomach to tighten. Her parents came to recognize that while Josh can tolerate a high level of pressure and perform well, Sara does best with lots of encouragement, getting things done early, studying in a quiet room, and taking frequent breaks.

Interpreting Pain Signals

When it comes to pain, interpretation and context have turned out to be much more important than first thought to be. Biology, neurology, physiology, and genetics are all very important, but what about our psychological interpretation of what pain means to us? The story we tell ourselves about our painful experiences influences the pain signal, opening or closing the pain gate. At age thirty-nine, Dr. Del Pozo slid into second base during a softball game. With adrenaline pumping, she did not feel the pain of scrapes and gravel stuck to her legs—especially because she was called safe! She was happy to sacrifice a little skin for the team. (It helped to win the game, too.) Imagine if she had been tagged out, lost the game, or, worse, if someone had tripped her! She interpreted the scrapes as a necessary sacrifice and badge of honor—when she finally did notice them.

That was an acute injury, at worst. With chronic pain, it is even more important to be aware of how we are interpreting the pain signals. With each tummy twinge or surge of nausea before an exam, if we interpret it as dangerous—"This is horrible! I can't do this! What if I have an accident? Something is terribly wrong!"—it is likely to increase. If instead we understand and think, "There's that tightness again. I must be feeling a little anxious, which is normal for me before an exam," then we are likely not to overinterpret the pain signal to mean more than it does. This is neuroplasticity in action.

A Multi-Directional Model for the Exacerbation of IBS Symptoms

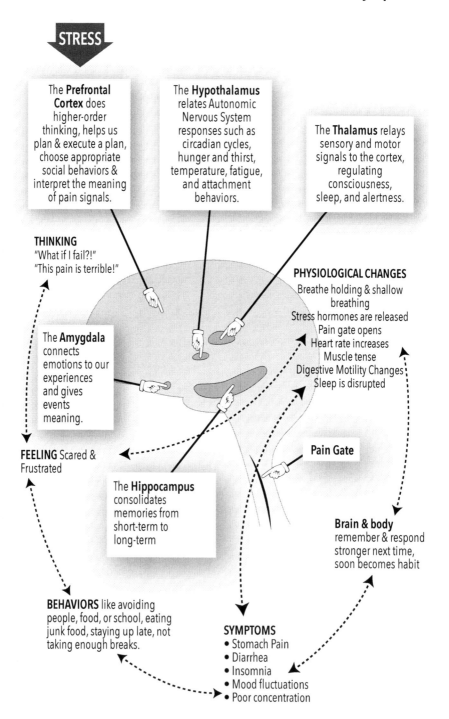

STRESS

The **Prefrontal Cortex** does higher-order thinking, helps us plan & execute a plan, choose appropriate social behaviors & interpret the meaning of pain signals.

The **Hypothalamus** relates Autonomic Nervous System responses such as circadian cycles, hunger and thirst, temperature, fatigue, and attachment behaviors.

The **Thalamus** relays sensory and motor signals to the cortex, regulating consciousness, sleep, and alertness.

THINKING
"What if I fail?!"
"This pain is terrible!"

PHYSIOLOGICAL CHANGES
Breathe holding & shallow breathing
Stress hormones are released
Pain gate opens
Heart rate increases
Muscle tense
Digestive Motility Changes
Sleep is disrupted

The **Amygdala** connects emotions to our experiences and gives events meaning.

FEELING Scared & Frustrated

Pain Gate

The **Hippocampus** consolidates memories from short-term to long-term

Brain & body remember & respond stronger next time, soon becomes habit

BEHAVIORS like avoiding people, food, or school, eating junk food, staying up late, not taking enough breaks.

SYMPTOMS
• Stomach Pain
• Diarrhea
• Insomnia
• Mood fluctuations
• Poor concentration

Our situation and genetics can predispose us to certain problems; however it is our perception and management of stress that predicts how good we feel and how well we function day-to-day.

CHAPTER SUMMARY

- The journey from food to poop is long and includes the digestive tract, commanded by the brain. It involves the immune system and a multitude of messages between the brain and the gut.

- Accommodation is the automatic adjustment the stomach and intestines make for food. This accommodation system is dysfunctional in people with IBS.

- The pain gate allows messages of discomfort to be turned up (open gate) or down (closed gate), causing more or less pain to be perceived. People with IBS feel pain at a lower threshold. This is partially due to more messages going through an open gate and being interpreted by the frontal lobe as bad.

- Stressful events open the pain gate and increase pain, while calming or enjoyable activities close the gate and reduce pain.

- Our subjective interpretation of pain brings meaning to it, for better or worse. We can change the story and reroute neurons. This is because of the neuroplasticity of the brain.

? QUESTIONS FOR YOUR FAMILY

Each family member can take a turn answering the following questions.

1) What is the story you tell yourselves about IBS?

2) What events were in place when it began? What was the situation during the most recent flare-up?

CHAPTER 3

Building Confidence about the Diagnosis

How is IBS Diagnosed?

I BS is frustrating—to say the least—for the patient, the patient's family, the doctor, and the health care system. Some are frustrated just trying to nail down a diagnosis, while others are discouraged with the diagnosis itself, as it does not lend itself to open-the-hood-and-fix-it sort of doctoring.

Many parents agonize that something else is terribly wrong that doctors just have not found yet (and all this worrying makes the IBS worse!). Doctors become frustrated not knowing what else to do (no one likes feeling helpless). It doesn't help that just like a migraine headache, IBS does not show up in any objective measures such as blood tests, imaging, biopsies, or endoscopies. Although it may seem old-fashioned, the best way to diagnose someone with IBS is by listening to and looking at the person. IBS can be diagnosed correctly 96 percent of the time by symptoms, rule-outs, and the overall clinical picture.

Symptoms of IBS include three months or more of continuous or recurrent:

- Stomach pain or discomfort;
- Diarrhea and/or constipation; or
- Other digestive symptoms, such as vomiting, gas, or bloating.

The problem lies with the function of the bowels and is therefore called a "functional" disorder (rather than a disease). The good news is that there is no organic disease process occurring (such as infection), and having IBS does not put you at higher risk for digestive diseases later (such as inflammatory bowel disease or cancer). It is easy to fall into the trap of going on a mission for "the real cause," passing right by the obvious (think forest-trees scenario). Using fancy scans or scopes will not help identify IBS any better, and, as we have said, more invasive procedures can lead to more problems. If a school-aged child has tummy aches, some diarrhea or constipation perhaps, maybe problems sleeping, and a headache or three, there is a very good chance he or she has IBS. Other telltale signs include a downtrodden or listless look mixed with a bit of shame. The stress children with IBS carry is palpable. The isolation and alienation that IBS brings has just started to take root.

Parents Often Ask, "What Else Could It Be?"

You may still be wondering if your child really has IBS. You may have lost confidence in doctors and fear that they missed something. We can shine some light on this, realizing, of course, that it is no substitute for a working relationship with your pediatrician.

Here are the problems that need to be ruled out before a diagnosis of IBS is concluded:

1) Crohn's Disease

2) Ulcerative Colitis

3) Celiac Sprue

Crohn's disease is one type of inflammatory bowel disease that can affect all layers of the intestinal mucosa anywhere from mouth to anus. Crohn's can result in partial bowel obstruction, bleeding, and malabsorption. This autoimmune condition is rare, affecting around twelve people per one hundred thousand every year, with higher rates in people who have a family member with Crohn's. Crohn's can masquerade for some time but typically it rears its ugly head as:

- Pain

- Vomiting

- Weight loss

- Failure to thrive, or

- Anemia

Sometimes there is associated joint swelling, eye inflammation, skin abnormalities, and mouth ulcers. A complete blood count and a C reactive protein test will indicate that there is a problem that requires further investigation.

Ulcerative colitis is another type of inflammatory bowel disease that affects only the top layer of mucosa that lines the large intestine and rectum. Ulcerative colitis occurs in twenty-four persons per one hundred thousand every year, and is also more common when another family member has it. Ulcerative colitis presents with:

- Diarrhea—usually bloody and often painless

- Joint swelling and

- Skin problems (occasionally)

Ulcerative colitis can be identified with blood and stool tests that detect inflammation in the intestines.

Celiac sprue is an immune response to the gluten protein found in wheat. An enzyme called tissue transglutaminase modifies the gluten protein while the immune system cross-reacts with the small-bowel tissue. The inflammatory result leads to a truncating of the villi (tiny fiber-like projections) that line the small intestine. This interferes with the absorption of nutrients, as the intestinal villi are responsible for absorption. The only known effective treatment is a lifelong gluten-free diet. While the disease is caused by a reaction to wheat proteins, it is not the same as a wheat allergy.

Gluten is a protein found in wheat, oats, barley, and rye. People with celiac disease may present with varying symptoms, but they usually have diarrhea and signs of poor absorption of nutrients, since the condition only affects the small bowel (where nutrients are absorbed). The current blood test for celiac sprue is very sensitive but produces incorrect or "false positive" results in up to 30 percent of patients. Therefore, further tests may be needed to confirm the diagnosis before committing to a lifelong restrictive diet. A celiac sprue diagnosis can be made first by a screening blood test, then by biopsy of the small intestine.

Celiac sprue may affect up to one in two hundred persons; however, a recent study from the Mayo Clinic showed that it is no more common in people with IBS than in the normal population. Many people with IBS believe they have celiac sprue because they feel better when they avoid gluten. One study showed that 30 percent of people with IBS proven not to have celiac sprue felt significantly better on a wheat-free diet. This may imply that avoiding wheat products in general during an IBS flare may help, but a rigid gluten-free diet is not necessary or advised.

Other Things It's Not

Wheat Sensitivity

Gluten-sensitive people who have IBS do not demonstrate the so-called "leaky gut" permeability of celiac sprue and colitis that indicates a separation in epithelial cells (cells that layer organs) in the intestines. So why do they feel better when avoiding wheat products? A good explanation can be found in the constituents of fermentable fructans that exist in wheat products, whose byproducts are chemicals (such as alcohols and ketones) that may affect gastrointestinal function and sensitivity. Normal fermentation in the colon produces gas that may be difficult for people with IBS to tolerate because of visceral hypersensitivity and altered transit of food. Therefore, the benefits of a gluten-free diet may be the consequence of less fermentation in the colon. Some research has shown that many people who thought they had gluten sensitivity did not improve with wheat or gluten elimination. When challenged with wheat alone, only about 2 percent of IBSers developed symptoms.

Food Allergies

Food allergies are usually an immune response to a food protein. The immite system misidentifies the food as an invader and responds by attacking it. Food allergies tend to be most prevalent in the first few years of life, affecting 6 percent of infants less than three years of age. Nutritional tolerance to many of the dietary proteins often improves with age and children outgrow the allergy. But if not, these children must avoid the trigger food to avoid the allergic reaction, which may be mild to severe and even life threatening.

When testing people with IBS for food allergies, the results have shown that IBSers tend to overestimate the prevalence of food allergies, especially when using questionnaire-based diagnosis. This is a common mistake since food seems to be the culprit in a digestive-related disorder. However, allergies that have acute life-threatening and anaphylactic responses start within one hour of ingestion of the food. These foods may affect skin, lungs, or the gastrointestinal tract. An extreme allergic reaction to food is rarely connected to IBS. When true food allergies do occur, they are usually due to cow's milk or wheat products and occasionally egg, soy, or nuts. Parents often discover this by introducing one food at a time to the infant. Skin prick and blood tests for sensitivities have proven unreliable. Unless it is a clear food allergy, very restrictive elimination diets are usually not healthy and can lead to food neurosis (control and anxiety problems) and sometimes anorexia-like conditions. Typically, for IBS, the stress level of the gut and the way food is ingested predict symptoms better than which type of food is eaten. When food seems to exacerbate IBS, it is often due to exaggerated stomach-to-colon (gastrocolic) reflex and psychological distress.

Lactose Malabsorption (Intolerance)

Twenty percent of the population tests positive for lactose malabsorption, which means these people lack the enzyme or have insufficient levels of lactase needed to break down lactose into simple sugars to be absorbed by the gut. The lactose that escapes absorption in the small intestine becomes fermented to hydrogen gas in the large bowel. The relation of lactose malabsorption to chronic stomach pain and gas is unclear. In other words, the amount of hydrogen gas produced in lactose malabsorption does not predict who has gas or pain. Also, consumption of lactose with a meal (rather than alone) can seemingly reduce the crampy effects of malabsorbed lactose. There are other modifying factors as well, such as the rate the stomach and small bowel move food contents along, effects of bacteria genotypes in the colon, and, perhaps most importantly, individual visceral hypersensitivity. The 20 percent of people who are lactose intolerant likely avoid the dairy products that bother them and do not have other digestive problems unless they also have IBS.

A recent study of IBSers in Spain showed that self-reported lactose intolerance at home was far more frequent than could be predicted by a lactose breath test, which is considered the gold standard for lactose malabsorbtion. In fact, only half the self-reported malabsorbers who thought they suffered from lactose intolerance had a positive lactose hydrogen breath test to prove it. These findings leave many people confused as to whether or not they should eat dairy products, which ones, and how much.

The conclusion from the Spanish study was that lactose malabsorption was a relatively minor contributor to the symptoms for people with IBS, even though many people attributed their symptoms to consumption of dairy products. This study emphasized the contribution of the home environment regarding diet and stress to be more important. For the same reason, offending food is often better tolerated on a relaxing vacation. Hospital staff have observed this phenomenon in highly symptomatic IBS patients who make miraculous recoveries when admitted to hospital—often a more supportive and nurturing environment than that from whence they came.

Although lactose may be overly blamed for IBS flares, many adults do lose the lactase enzyme with age. Dairy products may also seem like a trigger food for IBS because of the amount of inherent sugar they contain, or simply because the large size of the casein molecule in dairy is more difficult to digest. (Corn, soy, and wheat gluten are also considered oversized molecules.) These foods may be generally more difficult for a sensitive stomach to digest in large quantities. Considering all these factors, people with IBS may choose to limit high-lactose products (like low-fat milk) and other foods with oversized molecules. However, dairy products do contribute important nutrients, such as calcium and vitamin D, and should not be "demonized" or restricted without good cause.

The Bacterial Overgrowth Hypothesis

An overgrowth of gut bacteria happens when the flora of the gut changes significantly and bad bacteria take over and prevent absorption of necessary nutrients. This condition is extremely rare; yet bacteria overgrowth is often blamed for IBS symptoms. Some people even take a breath test to "prove" it; however, these tests are very inconsistent. At the same time, gut bacteria are a fascinating frontier in medical research, and the health of our gut flora is directly connected to our overall health.

Bacteria in the large intestine comprise 70 percent of all the body's cells. There are over one thousand different species, yet only a third of these have been identified. Think of intestinal bacteria like our universe—exploration is in its infancy. There are two gut ecosystems, one inside the intestinal lumen (tube) and one on the mucosal lining of the intestine. The bacteria play a significant role in the health of the mucosa as well as intestinal immune function, motility, gut permeability, and sensitivity. Diet, antibiotics, and probiotics can temporarily alter the bowel's ecology, but it rapidly returns to baseline.

Post-Infectious IBS

Nearly 30 percent of IBSers are convinced that their symptoms began after an acute gastrointestinal illness. Although this may seem true, it is more likely that the original infection simply uncovered or triggered the IBS, allowing it to surface. Meanwhile, other factors, such as anxiety, perpetuate the chronic digestive problems. After a gastroenteritis outbreak in Canada from water contamination, IBS symptoms were four times more likely to be present in persons infected during a time of psychological distress (e.g., divorce, job loss). Over time, the symptoms in these people tend to wane even though it may take months to years.

It Still Has to Be "Something Else"

We often hear concerns from our patients that they still fear the doctor missed something. Parents often believe their child's IBS is more than a chronic, nonfatal, functional problem. Sometimes this is because of the psychological stigma attached to IBS in the medical community that it is not a "real" and valid medical problem. This erroneous belief along with others lead people to mistakenly reject an accurate diagnosis of IBS. We have helped many families move forward from these beliefs that were keeping them stuck. Here are some of the most common "sticky points" below:

1) Many people who suffer a lot of pain believe that something terrible or fatal must be wrong, or it just does not make sense.

2) Many people want something more "curable" to be wrong so they can quest forward to the cure. It is frustrating to hear "you may have to manage this for the rest of your life" instead of "here, take this pill."

3) Many people feel their doctors do not listen to them and lump their symptoms into a patronizingly nebulous "catchall" diagnosis; they therefore are not satisfied with the diagnosis received. This is especially common with problems diagnosed without tests to validate the source of pain.

4) Some people do not want a diagnosis that is stress related, assuming that this means they have been told it is "all in their head" and they are certainly above "all that."

5) Often people with IBS have general anxiety as well as anxiety about IBS, so continued worry even after a proper diagnosis is common.

6) It is not easy to make the necessary lifestyle changes to feel better with IBS; therefore, not accepting the diagnosis is a way to avoid this challenging endeavor.

7) Related to # 6, accepting a diagnosis of IBS may force some people to examine the stress in their lives more carefully, and this can be difficult or painful.

We followed over 200 children with IBS for over three years after the inception of the SEEDS program and found that the referring physician got the correct diagnosis—every time. No organic diseases surfaced later that had been misidentified. Accepting the diagnosis of IBS is key to moving forward to manage it successfully. There is a lot that we do understand about IBS, and we will share what we know with you. The current scientific information supports that one single predominant mechanism is unlikely. Multiple mechanisms likely operate simultaneously, making a multimodal approach and a critical yet open mind imperative.

CHAPTER SUMMARY

- It is common for someone with IBS to be worried that something else is the problem and doctors have missed it.

- It is unlikely that you have something other than IBS if your doctor has performed a thorough exam.

- The common conditions your doctor will rule out include Crohn's disease, ulcerative colitis, and celiac sprue. These diseases are typically diagnosed with blood tests.

- Food allergies, lactose intolerance, and gluten sensitivities are overestimated in the IBS population; however, reducing these foods may minimize symptoms for other reasons (like reducing fructans).

- Bacterial overgrowth is likely unrelated to IBS; however, a healthy gut flora is important.

- Many people notice IBS begins after an acute infection, but symptoms are likely perpetuated by psychological distress in a sensitive gut rather than due to the original infection.

- Acceptance of the diagnosis is key to moving forward toward minimizing symptoms and flare-ups of IBS.

chapter 4

CHAPTER 4

Treatments: The Good, the Bad, the Failed

Traditional Tests and Treatments

I n these days of modern medicine with high-tech machines and incredible procedures, patients can be left with the expectation that everything can and should be fixed, if only they could find and afford the latest high-tech medical treatment. Many people feel they have been undertreated when in fact they have been overtreated. More is not always better—a notion that remains generally unsupported by the American lifestyle.

Medical care providers have a responsibility to carefully weigh the pros and cons of tests and procedures. Patients also have a role in taking responsibility for their health. As patients, we may not pay enough attention to our own health sometimes, but other times may overinterpret the importance of a symptom. Overinterpretation of the significance of a relatively minor symptom is called "catastrophizing" and often leads to inappropriate tests and overtreatment, which can lead to more problems. Doctors and patients need to work together to hear and understand each other to maximize health and quality of life. We will review common traditional treatments for IBS, including doctor visits, surgeries, scans, and medications, and then review complementary and alternative therapies used for IBS.

49

Doctor Visits

Primary care doctors often feel frustrated because they cannot cure IBS and hence have a sense of inadequacy. Emergency physicians often consult surgeons who have little experience with functional pain syndromes, so they both sometimes fail to recognize the pain for what it is—an exacerbation of a chronic disorder. Prescriptions are often given to placate IBSers even when the practitioner knows there is unlikely to be any long-term benefit after the placebo effect has worn off. The placebo effect for medications is often quite high, and even higher for surgeries. However, the effects eventually wear off and symptoms return. Meanwhile, the underlying issues related to stress go unattended.

Surgeries

Avoiding unnecessary procedures is important, especially when there is a good amount of certainty that there is no organic disease pathology. Many people with IBS have been found to have normal appendixes after urgent appendectomies. We now know that gallbladder surgeries and hysterectomies are much more likely to be done on IBSers, resulting in significant cost, suffering, and even death. People who catastrophize (believe something is far worse than it is) after surgery have more anxiety, leading to higher visceral hypersensitivity and more pain, which can lead, again, to more parts being unnecessarily removed.

Colonoscopies and Computed Tomography (CT) Scans

Parents often request a colonoscopy for their children, driven by the fear of missing a disease. However, more than one thousand IBSers undergoing colonoscopy showed no greater incidence of pathology, such as Crohn's disease or Ulcerative Colitis. IBS is not a diagnosis made just by exclusion. IBS can be confidently identified in the office at the time of the first visit after taking a careful history and examination, and in the absence of warning signs like weight loss, bleeding from the GI tract, anemia, or family history of celiac disease or inflammatory bowel disease.

Tests carry risks. CT scans increase your risk of cancer with radiation exposure over the course of a lifetime. Reproductive organs and breast tissue are particularly radiosensitive. Other effects can be allergic reaction and renal failure from the dye. A CT scan is rarely helpful as a diagnostic tool for people with non-acute abdominal pain, but is commonly reported to show incidental, or "red herring," abnormalities that do not explain the pain. This often results in more anxiety and more specialty referrals, additional imaging procedures, and surgeries that do not help the patient.

Emergency physicians and surgeons focus on excluding acute organic illness by ordering more lab tests and radiological exams. When we looked at children with IBS four years after SEEDS, they are four times less likely to have radiological exams. This is in part because we educated the parents about unnecessary tests for their children, sparing medical staff and expense, but, most of all, sparing children from unnecessary tests.

Medications

Only a third of all medications given to people with IBS are gastrointestinal medications. The remaining two thirds are for the co-morbid diagnoses, such as migraine headaches or fibromyalgia. We see children on opiate painkillers (Vicodin, Norco, morphine, and others), which are the worst treatments that can be given for IBS. Not only do opiate painkillers not provide a solution, but a primary side effect is constipation. Also, the body naturally habituates to opiates over time, requiring higher levels of opiates to reach the same amount of pain relief. This can lead to the trap of taking more and more, causing other health problems or impairment.

Although medication trials are expensive to run, over 90 percent of the research and development dollars are spent on advertising to you via commercials, such as the ones telling you to "ask your doctor." This has left a vast and erroneous belief that there are effective medications for most ailments. In general, it is wise to be skeptical of medication trials sponsored by pharmaceutical companies when the investigators have a financial benefit from the outcome.

IBSers have been given antibiotics in the belief that they have an excess of bacteria in their small bowel, but very few benefit from them. The trials with antibiotics in adults have produced minor improvements in symptoms, mainly by reducing gas and bloating. Only a few patients had long-term benefit. Many of us working in the trenches have rarely seen "cures" with this approach, and a trial of the broad-spectrum antibiotic Rifaximin failed to improve symptoms compared to placebos for children. Long-term antibiotics can also make symptoms worse by disrupting the gut flora even more. Antibiotics do not discriminate well between the good and bad bacteria, so they kill off the good bacteria with the bad.

Laxatives for Constipation

When we feel the urge to defecate (poop), our rectum straightens, going from a 90 percent angle to 120 percent, allowing waste to descend. We can control our anal sphincter (the outlet valve) by voluntarily squeezing or tightening. If we are ready to go and the rectum is straight, then we relax the sphincter. When things are working well, all of this happens automatically. Problems with constipation and fecal retention can start at a young age and are more common that you might think. Up to 20 percent of children have functional defecation disorders. It may start with a child not wanting to stop playing to go to the bathroom, and this sets up the withholding cycle. More commonly, the withholding starts after an experience of a hard, painful, or frightening bowel movement. Low fiber, inadequate fruit and vegetable intake, obesity, and family history contribute to it.

Retained or withheld stools become more difficult to move, and a vicious fear-avoidance cycle begins with hard stools too painful to pass. Continued fecal retention is like a dam across a rising river—eventually it overflows, leading to fecal incontinence or spurious diarrhea and soiling of underwear. Children (and adults) become terribly embarrassed and isolated and may ultimately lose their urge to defecate as the act of pooping becomes linked to feeling bad.

Untreated, functional defecation disorders can persist for years. Sadly, chronic constipation in childhood tends to persist into adulthood and is a predictor of adult IBS. The best therapy is disimpaction (removing the poop with oral laxatives) and behavioral therapy for the bowels (using the bathroom regularly). Maintenance of regular defecation is important to prevent relapse of constipation and may be needed for months to years. Soluble fiber (such as Psyllium husk) works for some people, while probiotics do not help constipation. Polyethylene glycol, or Miralax, the "master blaster," may also help maintain regular bowel function once the bowel is clean. Then, reinforce spontaneous use of the toilet with small rewards (especially after breakfast), and always have the child wear clean underwear. Teach him about his anatomy and instruct him how to strain and how to withhold stool.

Complementary and Alternative Medicine

Complementary and alternative medicine (CAM) is a diverse group of medical treatments that are not usually considered part of conventional Western medicine. Many CAM treatments come from ancient Eastern practices that are known for emphasizing context and multiple causes affecting health, as opposed to a stricter biological cause-effect model. Many patients combine CAM treatments with Western medical treatment, including up to half of people with IBS. CAM treatments encompass several categories: natural products, mind-body medicines, and manipulative body-based practices.

Natural Products

Herbs

Natural products include herbal medicines, peppermint oil, exclusion diets, probiotics, and prebiotics. There have been four studies so far showing the following herbal supplements helpful for IBS: Chinese herbal medicines (TCM), Tibetan herbal formula (Padma Lax), and two complex extracts of herbs (STW5 and STW 5-11). At follow-up three months later, only the patients in the TCM group who received individualized treatments continued to show improvement. Like many treatments for IBS, they worked briefly, but did not help long term. Authenticating the active ingredients is another challenge of using supplements.

Peppermint

Peppermint oil is a smooth muscle relaxant, or carmative, commercially

available in enteric coated capsules designed to deliver the active ingredients into the large intestines. Some studies have shown benefits, and the
active ingredients seem safe. In 1988, one of the authors (Dr. Lawson)
published a placebo-controlled study of enteric-coated peppermint oil—
meaning the real peppermint ingredient was compared to a supplement
with no active ingredient. Both peppermint and the placebo worked well,
so although some people find peppermint helps, it is still not widely used
(neither is placebo as a treatment). If you do decide to try peppermint
capsules, be forewarned that side effects can include rectal irritation and
minty-smelling flatulence.

Probiotics and Prebiotics

Some research supports the idea that the gastrointestinal bacteria community is disturbed in IBS patients. It is unclear whether this contributes
as a causal factor of IBS symptoms or a byproduct of the central nervous
system disruption. However, some experts believe that the disturbed gut
bacteria phenomenon leads to low-grade inflammation, hypersensitivity
to gut pain, and hypercontractility.

Probiotics are microorganisms, not strictly alive, that are a component of human microflora in the gut. They are acid resistant and can
usually be recovered in the stool. Probiotics are thought to decrease inflammation, improve gut barrier function (permeability) and improve
the threshold at which we feel sensations. Although microflora changes
with probiotics have been inconsistent, there have been some significant
responses to the probiotic Bifidobacterium infantis, which seems to improve abdominal pain. Another type of probiotic, VSL #3 (freeze-dried
lactic acid bacteria), has also been shown to reduce flatulence and bloating in adults. A recent adolescent crossover trial (using patients as their
own control) showed a small but statistically significant improvement in
overall symptom severity and perception of pain and bloating.

Probiotics may help normalize the bacteria colonies in the intestines
and improve an IBSer's quality of life by reducing gas and bloating. There
is also some evidence that prebiotics—another dietary supplement—may
improve stool consistency, flatulence, and bloating.

Studies in bacteria-free animals suggest a link between probiotics and control of gastric emptying, abnormal intestinal transit times, intestinal permeability, and visceral sensation, although a cause-effect relationship has yet to be established. Some of these experimental changes appear to normalize with the use of probiotics.

Probiotics may help a little by improving the good bacteria, but what about killing off the bad bacteria? Helicobacter pylori (H. pylori) can cause a gastric bacterial infection that is more prevalent among people who have dyspepsia or indigestion. In the past, eradication of the bacteria with antibiotics has been advocated as a treatment for individuals with functional dyspepsia. Despite a recent study in Brazil showing a 12.5 percent improvement beyond placebo, there has been reduced enthusiasm for antibiotic treatment, primarily because of the adverse events such as bacteria-resistant strains and toxins associated with antibiotic therapy—without clear and long-lasting clinical benefit.

Fecal Infusions

There is a more extreme treatment called fecal microbiota transplantation, or fecal infusion, which has revolutionized the management of a debilitating intestinal infection known as Clostridium difficle (C. diff). This evil overgrowth usually occurs in susceptible individuals who are taking antibiotics—often those in long-term care facilities or hospitals. The normal intestinal flora is temporarily suppressed, allowing the C. diff to take over producing a toxin that causes severe and sometimes fatal diarrhea. A rather innovative treatment of fecal infusion that includes infusing feces from a normal person into the colon of a recurrent C. diff sufferer has a 90 percent chance of sustained cure. Canadian researchers have produced an artificial culture of normal colonic flora to be as close as possible to real gut flora. Early results look promising for C. diff and the product will be known as "Repoopulate." The lessons to learn here are: 1) your gut flora is there to protect you from disease, and 2) don't take antibiotics unless absolutely necessary. There may be a role for this approach in some IBS patients, but it is much too early to tell. (Finding a stinky placebo for a randomized, blinded trial is one challenge.)

Acupuncture

Acupuncture is based on the theory that internal energy (chi) runs through meridians, or channels. Disruption of chi energy is thought to contribute to symptoms. Bodily functions can be manipulated by activating these meridians with penetration of thin, solid metallic needles. Acupuncture is thought to lower visceral hypersensitivity and motility by stimulating the parasympathetic nervous system and the vagus nerve, thus altering the brain-gut axis. However, current evidence does not support the use of acupuncture for treatment of IBS. Both acupuncture and sham (placebo) acupuncture improve IBS symptoms. However, we can learn much from CAM therapies as they focus on an individualized, holistic approach with attention to the patient's physiological needs and coping difficulties.

The Placebo Effect

A placebo effect is actual or perceived improvement for a medical condition despite there being no active treatment ingredient present. Treatment studies without comparison of the real treatment to a blinded placebo (control) group should be reviewed with skepticism. The efficacy of placebo in IBS can reach up to 80 percent and is typically around 30–40 percent. In 2010, in a study called "placebo without deception," patients were given these placebo pills and told the truth, that indeed it contained only nonactive ingredients; yet, their symptoms still improved. The IBS patients in this study taking the placebo pills showed a 60 percent improvement, which approaches the demonstrated benefit of so-called "active" medications in controlled trials. Children with IBS show such a high placebo response, making it less likely that any drug will be able to show a significant benefit over and above placebo treatment.

What does this strong placebo response tell us? Perhaps the individual attention provided during drug studies, the belief that help is on the way, the hope for relief, and validation that something is being done all have a powerful effect on human central operating mechanisms (brain and spinal cord), even (or perhaps especially) if unconscious. After learning this, patients and medical providers alike ask, "Shouldn't we all take placebos then?" This is an interesting question with many layers up for debate.

CHAPTER SUMMARY

Some of the traditional treatments—such as doctor and emergency room visits, CT scans, and certain medications—have generally been found to be ineffective for IBS. In fact, unnecessary tests can carry their own risks and also distract people from dealing with important issues such as stress.

There is some evidence to suggest that probiotics, fiber, laxatives, and some herbal supplements may help some people manage certain symptoms of IBS.

chapter 4

PART II

Planting the SEEDS

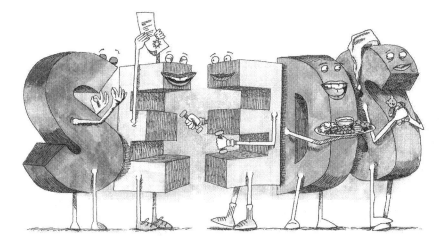

CHAPTER 5

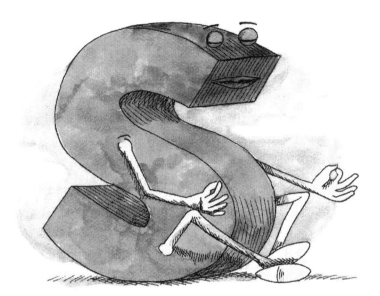

SEEDS: Stress and Calming the Central Nervous System

The first S in SEEDS stands for stress management. In this chapter we will:

- Identify stress that children experience.

- Understand the IBS-stress relationship.

- Observe thoughts and beliefs that can contribute to or alleviate symptoms.

- Learn about emotions and how to handle them.

- Manage stress better with eighteen stress busters.

- Acknowledge the media's influence on our daily lives.

What's Stress Got To Do With It, Really?

"Is my child's IBS just stress?" No, not *just* stress, which makes the role of stress sound less important than it really is. Stress is much more than just stress. Our brains are constantly scanning our surroundings to see what danger may be lurking. They can go into protective mode quite easily. When our brains perceive fear, the fight-flight-freeze response is triggered. Heart rate increases, as do blood pressure and breathing rate. Muscles tense and digestion ability decreases as blood rushes toward the heart, lungs, and large muscle groups. Cortisol and other stress hormones are dumped into the blood stream. More specifically, corticotrophin-releasing factor is involved in stress-induced changes in intestinal motility and mucosal barrier function. Diarrhea is one way to get rid of extra work for the body during a stressful time. Slowing digestion with constipation is another option that allows precious resources to temporarily be rerouted elsewhere. Many people suffer alternating diarrhea and constipation along with stomach upset.

So what does stress have to do with the digestive tract? Actually, everything. Your guts and your gut reaction are directly related to what your brain perceives as dangerous. It does not matter if there is actual danger; your guts will respond the same whether the danger is truly there or not. This is all in order to prepare your body for action if necessary. Over time, the preparing-for-action system becomes very tired and starts to disregulate, causing physical and emotional symptoms. This stress-induced fight-flight-freeze response varies throughout the day—often below our awareness. (Observe your body the next time you drive past a state trooper, even when you are not breaking the law.)

Our brains (frontal lobes and amygdalas especially) perceive and interpret information into thoughts and sensations that lead us to behave in certain ways, for better or worse. When we perceive something as uncomfortable or scary, it affects our bodily sensations, as well as how we choose to respond. One person may perceive airplane travel as exciting, while another perceives it as scary. The one who finds it exciting might get goose bumps or feel energized while packing for a trip. The one who finds it scary may become nauseous just thinking about the airport and avoid air travel altogether. Each one has a different reaction and decides to do something different based on feelings and beliefs (this is fun versus this is horribly unsafe). Once a situation has been deemed unsafe, the central nervous system quickly encodes this. It may then become hardwired, and we start generalizing to other situations.

Emotion	Situation	Thought & Belief	Physiological Response	Behavior	Generalized Behavior
FEAR	Difficult Math Test	I Am Not Prepared I'm a Failure	Stomach Upset	Avoid Test	Avoid School

The most basic way to undo the hardwiring and calm the nervous system is to learn one or two relaxation techniques that work for you and then use them daily. The children who come in for the relaxation portion of SEEDS are a bit nervous and not terribly interested in being told how to breathe or what to visualize. But within twenty minutes, they are so relaxed it sometimes takes them a few minutes to wake up enough to get off the floor! Relaxation is a natural state for the body, but one we have unlearned somewhere along the way and need to relearn now.

Tap into Your Healing Response: Introduction to Diaphragmatic Breathing

Diaphragmatic breathing retraining, visualization, and progressive muscle relaxation are relaxation techniques that help your body move from the stress response to the healing response. They are simple techniques once you learn them, but often underestimated in their ability to help us heal. Slowing your breath also slows your heart rate and blood pressure, helps improve blood flow to your digestive tract, and helps you process and absorb food better. Diaphragmatic breathing works best when you practice it regularly. You can start practicing for two minutes and add one minute each day until you reach twenty to thirty minutes. Your chest remains relatively still during this exercise, while your tummy does the breathing. Practice in a comfortable position in a safe place inside or outside. And don't underestimate the power of your breath!

Practice: Start out in a comfortable position, lying down or sitting with your feet on the floor. If it helps you relax and concentrate, allow your eyes to close. You will be breathing with your diaphragm, the muscle beneath your lungs. It may help if you place one hand on your belly during this exercise to alert your belly (not your chest) to do the breathing.

Start by noticing your breath. Bring your attention to your breath by simply observing it. Do not try to change it. Notice the breath flowing in…and out. Notice what the air feels like flowing in your nose, down into your lungs, and back up and out. If your mind wanders to something else, gently guide it back to your breathing. (It may be like herding cats, but that's OK.)

Begin reading this more slowly as you inhale. If it helps you concentrate, consider counting as you exhale. If you lose count, simply start again. Inhale, 1, 2, 3, 4, 5 (pause) and exhale, 5, 4, 3, 2, 1 (pause).

When you are ready, inhale through your nose and guide the breath down into your belly, allowing your belly to rise as you breathe in through your nose. Allow your belly to fall back into place as you exhale air through your mouth. Slowly. Gently. Slowly inhale, allowing your belly to expand, and slowly exhale as your belly relaxes. (Pause for several breaths or repeat this paragraph.)

When you are ready, extend the length of your exhale, slowing your breathing down. (Pause for two breaths.)

When you are ready, slow and lengthen your inhale. Now your breathing is slower, calmer. If you feel short of breath, stop this exercise and breathe at your normal pace.

If you can, slow the rhythm of your breath down even more. With each exhale, let go of any tension you are holding in your belly. Let it gently fill up with air again, and slowly exhale all tension. Notice how it might feel different from one moment to the next. Now, try less. What we mean is, don't turn this into a difficult event. Make it easier for yourself.

Scan your body from your face and neck to your shoulders, back, belly, arms, legs, and feet. If you notice any tension in those areas, inhale slowly, then exhale any tension you are holding. Take your time.

Now bring your attention back to your tummy as it gently rises and falls with your breathing. Let your tummy feel warm and relaxed. Feel warmth and safety. Enjoy this calm feeling. Take your time.

Notice how your body feels different now than it does normally or when you feel scared. Our tension levels tend to rise throughout the day. Think of regular, intentional relaxation as a way to bring yourself back to the baseline. Put another way, if your tension cup is half full in the morning and almost full by the afternoon, it won't take but a drop of water to make you feel overwhelmed or feel pain. However, if you continue to return to a half-full cup throughout the day, you will feel less stressed and able to handle more by the end of each day. Remember you can practice this for several minutes almost anywhere. Let it become a good friend to help you relax and heal each day.

Regular relaxation is a powerful way to gain control of your nervous system and gain control of your symptoms. Relaxation techniques, in conjunction with a deeper understanding of how to manage stress, can really help you on your way to keeping the whole family healthy. People who practice regular meditation or deep relaxation get fewer colds, have better brain connections, and reduce their risk for other diseases, such as heart disease and stroke. They also get better sleep and experience improved mood.

Thought Awareness

When we cannot avoid all things stressful, it is important to be aware how certain thoughts and beliefs (our perception of what is going on) impact our digestive tracts. For example, if Sara finds going to school causes anxiety and nausea, she will do her best to avoid going to school. School is not actually causing Sara's anxiety, but Sara's experience of school triggers her stomach to tighten, stress hormones to be released, and pain receptors to be activated, and the result is that she feels sick. It is only natural, then, for Sara to do whatever she can to avoid going to school. But avoiding school will not be good for her in the long run; therefore, it is important to provide her with the support to manage her fears and stomach pain. As Sara practices relaxation techniques, she still thinks about school, but her physiological reaction is calmer and she feels in more control of her response.

School is one place children feel stressed, but there are many things that can stress children out. Bringing awareness to their stressors is where we need to start to improve coping and find solutions to make life easier.

What Stressors Impact Children?

Stressful events in a child's life may be hard for adults to identify with, since it is the parent/guardian who has the lion's share of the responsibility for food, clothes, home, and other bills. You might wonder, "What can my child possibly be stressed about? I am the one with all the stress!" However, your child's stress about school is just as stressful to her as your responsibilities are to you. It may also be tempting to think about how stressful your own childhood was and how "easy" your child has it. While it may be true, it is not helpful to do this type of comparison. What she feels is real, and her body is responding accordingly.

There are certainly traumatic events that can shape a child's future, as well as daily life stressors that can have a severe impact on healthy development. Learning how to cope with stressful events is key for each child to know how to manage stress in a healthy way now and in the future. Everybody has stress to varying degrees and different physiological and social resources available to cope with the cards he or she is dealt. Recognizing the potential sources of stress will help you better understand your child's experience.

Consider the following list of anxiety-provoking circumstances for children:

- Fighting or tension at home or in the marriage, even if it does not directly include your child.

- An absent parent: working long hours, divorce, separation, death.

- An ill parent: a child can feel afraid of losing a parent or become overly responsible for caring for an ill parent.

- Mixed messages from parents: when parents cannot agree about limits or discipline, it breeds confusion and chaos for children.

- An absent sibling: military, college, divorce, death, illness.

- Too much or the wrong type of responsibility: raising siblings, caregiving for an adult, or making adult-level decisions leads to a sense of responsibility that is inappropriate for children.

- Being overly controlled or criticized.

- Too much parental interference: pampering, micromanaging.

- Too little responsibility: lack of daily structure or routine that leads to lack of skill building and self-confidence, and breeds entitlement.

- Not enough parental guidance: being neglected or ignored, struggling to find his or her place in the family.

- Being overly coddled: reduced self-confidence and development of independence.

- Television: some TV shows can increase fears or encourage unrealistic expectations, adding to social pressures or simply over-stimulating children.

- Video games: some are violent, competitive, and reduce social development.

- Social pressure: fitting in at school and getting along with peers.

- Athletic performance pressure: pressure of competitive sports.

- Academic performance pressure: pressure of schoolwork.

- Loss of a grandparent or other caregiver.

- Loss of a pet.

- Chronic hurried schedules: overscheduled child, parent, or siblings.

- Anxiety or depression of a parent.

- Being compared to a sibling: competition, never feeling good enough.

- Anything that causes chaos: busy schedule, chaotic parenting where the rules change or are ambiguous and outcomes of behavior are not predictable.

- Change of any type: moving, changing schools, death in family.

- Feeling lonely, left out, alienated, misunderstood, or unnecessary.

Traumatic events may include emotional, physical, or sexual abuse, witnessing abuse or fighting among other family members, loss of a family member, a child's own illness or hospitalization, and moving away from friends or a familiar environment. Any of these stressors can cause a child to feel fearful, anxious, sad, angry, hopeless, or alone. There is no question that traumatic events impact the likelihood of medical problems over the course of a lifetime. Traumas alter the way that children's brains develop and record information. Even a single traumatic experience alters the brain's development. This is because of neuroplasticity, the ability of the brain to change as a result of one's experiences (see chapter 2). A traumatic event may be over, but changes have already taken place. Because the brain changes and the brain is the body's control center, traumas often manifest in physical symptoms throughout the entire body. However, with good support, the brain—no matter what age—can relearn and rewire its neural pathways. Neuroplasticity can produce impressive changes; it just seems harder once our brains are fully developed, which happens in our early twenties. (Yet former congresswoman Gabrielle Giffords made a remarkable comeback after being shot in the head.)

Daily life stressors can also impact a child's development and come in all shapes and sizes. There is chronic stress that accompanies perfectionism, an overscheduled household, interpersonal conflicts, and performance pressure. Performance pressure may be academic, social, or athletic. Pressure can be from one or both parents, spoken or unspoken, conscious or unconscious. A common shared anxiety is fear about how others perceive us. Children desperately want to fit in with their peers, and, even more, they want approval from their parents. Children naturally take on the expectations of their parents and try to live up to them. Sometimes they feel it is impossible and will give up trying out of fear of failure, while others continue pushing themselves and never feel it is good enough. One thing is for certain: your child will always seek to be accepted unconditionally by you.

A common shared anxiety is fear about how others perceive us.

Unconditional love for your child is no small feat. It sounds like it should be as natural as rain, but it is more like a hurricane at times. It takes a great deal of moment-to-moment awareness of your own issues to be fully present with your children, teaching and guiding them toward independence, knowing when to push and when to protect—all the while accepting them for exactly who they are.

Let's go back to Sara again for a moment. She feels most anxious when she is in the cafeteria at lunchtime, and the anxiety causes her to feel nauseous and sick to her stomach. To avoid this feeling, she avoids eating until he gets home; however, she is so hungry by then she gulps down any fast food she can find. This increases her dyspepsia (indigestion or heartburn), preventing her from focusing on homework and being able to fall asleep. This vicious cycle repeats itself, and Sara's beliefs that she cannot eat in public or eat much at all without pain become stronger. As she withdraws more socially, she feels more alone and hopeless about his situation.

Sara's parents helped her talk about the anxiety she had that, unbeknownst to them, started when they moved to a new neighborhood and school. She threw up the first day of school after eating lunch at the cafeteria, and since then has not been able to separate the fear of embarrassing herself and eating in public. At first, she was convinced it was food that was to blame. After talking about it with her mom and the school nurse, Sara realized it was anxiety that caused her stomach upset.

Sara and her mom arranged to practice relaxation skills in the nurse's office for ten minutes, followed by eating a small amount of her lunch there. Over a few weeks she was able to eat half of her lunch without feeling sick. During the weekends, Sara's parents invited a friend or two over for lunch for Sara to practice eating in a small, relaxed group. They had some setbacks along the way, but eventually Sara learned that when she felt anxious, she had the ability to calm her stomach down; and even if it was still a little nervous, slowly eating small amounts of food helped her feel better throughout the day.

When Anxiety and Depression Reach Critical Levels

Many children with IBS have anxiety severe enough to warrant professional treatment. Sometimes a little stress can cause an anxious child to develop chronic anxiety and can increase his or her risk for depression. Children with IBS are 30 percent more likely to commit suicide than children without IBS or psychiatric problems. This has to be taken seriously. This means talking to a health professional and following through with the appropriate care. Children with anxiety or depression are much more likely to become adults with anxiety, depression, and a host of other chronic health conditions. There is no shame in recognizing a problem and getting the best help you can. Not only is it a worthwhile investment; the true shame would be in having your child (and the rest of the family) suffer needlessly.

MANAGING STRESS

Identifying Emotions

Children often struggle to put what they are feeling into words. Emotions (like fear) can easily be confused with a thought ("I can't go to school") or a behavior (not going to school). Stating how we feel is not something we often practice, like baseball or arithmetic. It is likely that your child is more aware of the most recent movie star picked up for bad behavior than he is of his current emotional experience.

You can encourage growth of your child's emotional IQ by helping her identify feelings like happy, silly, tired, scared, sad, frustrated, angry, or confused. For example, when Sara would throw her books down after trying to figure out a math problem, her mom would check in to affirm her frustration and allow her some space to feel that way. It's OK to feel frustrated (it's the behaviors that can get us into trouble). Next time she would ask Sara how she was feeling and wait patiently for her to respond. You can set a tone to indicate that any and all emotions are acceptable (yes, even anger). Allow your children to feel the full spectrum of emotions and then teach them to manage emotions appropriately.

The important thing is that she is able express herself honestly (in words, not acting out or holding things in and feeling ill).

"What is frustrating about it?" her mother, Karen, asked her.

Sara sneered at her, then paused and said, "It seems like everything is so easy for Josh. It's not fair!"

Karen reflected back to Sara what she just said: "It feels terribly unfair that Josh does well in school, while you struggle sometimes."

"Yes!" Sara said. "Everything is easy for him. He is good at everything. Everyone likes him better."

Allowing her to express her frustration opened up a conversation about how Sara felt compared to her brother and believed he was favored. After Sara felt understood by her parents, they could help her see more clearly the things she excelled at. At first, her parents were tempted to take Sara's frustration personally as a criticism of how they support Sara and Josh differently. Sara's mother may have felt defensive and tried to convince her of how untrue it was, resulting in more emotional isolation for Sara. The safe environment for Sara to express herself emotionally allowed her parents to understand her better. Once she felt heard, she was open to ways her parents could help her move forward.

Connecting Emotions and Physical Sensations

Next, Sara practiced connecting thoughts and reactions to physical sensations. After some practice of putting words to how she felt, her mother asked her, "Where in your body do you feel that frustration right now?" This may seem silly at first. The typical response is, "Nowhere. I don't know," or "I feel it in my head. I have lots of thoughts." This is because we are accustomed to separating our minds and brains from our bodies. Over time, Sara learned to tune into where in the body she feels something tightening, tingling, tensing, hurting, burning, gurgling, racing, or perhaps quieting, calming, and releasing. Stress will often be felt in the stomach, but could be anywhere. Where specifically children feel they are holding stress is not as important as simply making the connection between what the brain is experiencing and the parallel physiological sensations.

Children have many seemingly irrational fears, but do not discourage them or suggest they are silly. By allowing them to experience even irrational fears, you are not encouraging them to become more anxious or fearful, but simply accepting what they are already feeling as real and important. Allow any difficult topic to be discussed, and resist the urge to fix problems immediately. And by all means do not try to talk them out of how they feel. Asking more questions in a matter-of-fact and concerned-interested tone will create a "we-are-in-this-together" feeling. Acknowledging your child's whole-being experience (mind and body) will set the stage for problem solving about what to do next. (We have noticed that parents who bring their children to SEEDS demonstrate their commitment to their children, and that intent contributes to the positive outcomes these children have.)

SITUATION

Sara's parents want her to play soccer after school. She does not want to because the bigger children on the team tease her about her small height and size.

THOUGHTS

"The team hates me. I am no good."

EMOTIONS

Sadness, rejection, fear, and humiliation.

BODY SENSATIONS

Tightness, stomach pain, headache, and diarrhea.

BEHAVIORS

Avoids eating with upset stomach, has difficulty concentrating at soccer practice, and withdraws from friends and activities.

SOLUTION

Help Sara express how she feels, bring awareness to the problem, and help her accept things she cannot change and focus on what she can (she cannot change her small stature, but can practice quickness and speed skills). Practice what she might say to the children teasing her (assertive communication). Let her decide what to do (increases her sense of control), which may include playing a noncompetitive sport instead.

Managing Emotions

Once Sara practiced expressing how she felt, her parents could guide her about how to respond to these emotions. Just because Sara feels scared of school does not necessarily mean she should stay home. Her parents reminded her it is OK to feel scared, frustrated, and angry. It is a normal part of life. (If someone tells you otherwise, he is selling something.) The same general principles apply to Josh. When he is angry with his sister, it does not mean he gets to hit her. Although avoidance and acting out aggressively are common responses to strong emotions, let your children know the other options available (such as direct communication) that will have more positive outcomes. Teach them about the natural consequences of their behavior (such as not doing homework on time and having twice as much for the weekend) or consequences that have been predetermined by you (such as telling a lie and losing phone privileges). Assist them in problem solving about other ways to manage frustration. Keep in mind, what works for one child may not necessarily work for another.

The Importance of Routine

Our bodies love routine. Just like babies, we do best with regular routines of sleeping and waking, eating, moving, and resting. Routine helps the body to prepare the proper hormones (like serotonin and tryptophan) for sleeping, as well as the right hormones for digestion (insulin and cholecystokinin). Even more importantly, knowing what to expect each day is important for your child to feel some sense of control in her life. When she knows to some degree what to expect, some anxieties can be laid to rest. Setting a good sleep-wake routine in place can also help you set up a successful eating routine, allowing the digestive system the comfort of knowing what to expect and to adapt to expected volume and content. (The same is true for the behavioral consequences set with consistent parenting discussed above.)

Knowing what to expect has been shown to be even more important than having plentiful resources like food. This was shown in several studies with monkeys. One group of monkeys was given a regular and plentiful supply of food, another group was given a regular but minimal amount of food, and the last group was given irregular amounts of food—often boun-

chapter 5

tiful amounts, but they were unpredictable. They never knew how much or when they would receive it. The behavior of the mother monkeys was different, depending on what group they were in. The groups who received regular amounts of food, even small amounts, demonstrated more loving behaviors than the group who received an erratic food supply. We humans, like monkeys, become much more stressed and irritable when we do not know what to expect. Routines do not have to be mundane; add variety and be flexible within a healthy structure.

> **Dr. Lawson** laughs the most watching his grandson Jack do almost anything. He is happy on a surfboard or skiing with his wife, Helen.
>
> **Dr. Del Pozo** laughs when her daughter Willow chases their chickens, and is most happy swinging in their hammock with Willow and her husband, Carlos. All three of them enjoy skiing with the Lawsons.

18 Stress Busters

There are many other ways to manage stress and reduce the tension around your house. Here are a few:

1) **Wake up ten minutes early**—yes, intentionally. Get ready first and use the extra time to relax, read, or talk before stepping out the door. This is difficult at first, but worth it.

2) **Meals and snacks should be eaten sitting down** in a relaxed environment, with upbeat conversation or peace and quiet.

3) **Get the least desirable homework/ housework done first** to get it out of the way.

4) When you are stuck somewhere waiting, use that time to **practice relaxation techniques** rather than becoming increasingly irritated. Take ownership of how you feel in these moments.

5) **Simplify your schedule.** Cut out unnecessary activities and organize daily activities using a large calendar that you and your child can fill in together. Include children in some of the planning, as appropriate for their developmental level.

6) **Use a reward chart** for tasks accomplished. Rewards could include items such as books or an outing with family or friends (picnic, movie).

7) **Stick with a routine,** but if the day goes awry, be flexible and let go of trying to control each event.

8) **Be prepared for days that just do not go as planned.** Have a backup plan that makes the most of unforeseen events.

9) Realize that when you are obsessing about something new, it is just an old habit directed at a new event (schoolwork, food, friends, parents). **Take a break from thinking about it.**

10) **Writing things down** always helps, whether or not you can even read your handwriting or whether or not you throw it away. It is the process of expressing yourself on paper that helps your brain relax.

11) Do not be afraid to **"be yourself."** What does that mean? Just be who you are at any given moment without trying to impress or please anyone else. Be honest about where you are at that moment (frustrated, tired, rejected).

12) **Respect each other,** even when you are stressed and tired, which means being *aware of when you are stressed and tired.*

13) **Get involved in noncompetitive sports.** Sports are great, but extra competition for a sensitive child may not be in his best interest at this time.

14) **Practice mindful eating.** Take your time, focus on the present moment, and enjoy each bite you are chewing.

15) **Observe your child's self-talk as well as your own.** Is he hard on himself? Is the talk negative sometimes? Are there negative messages you are reinforcing? (Don't blame yourself if you are; just learn from it.)

16) **Hold adult conversations** (your work stress, difficulties with your family, money, boss, politics, etc.) when your children are present.

17) Plan at least **one fun activity each day.**

18) **Laugh a lot!** Find out what makes you laugh and double the dose.

Media Influence

There has been controversy for many years about the impact of television (and other electronic media) on children. This can be a touchy topic with parents and children alike, so we will arm you with the facts and encourage common sense.

The National Television Violence Study (1994–1997) found two out of three television shows contained violence. Although violent television is not the primary cause of violence, it does increase aggressive behavior, fear, and acceptance of violent behavior. It also increases anxiety about becoming a victim of violence. Children who watch a lot of television also have lower grades, sleep poorly, are more obese, struggle more socially, have lower self-image, have fewer hobbies, use more alcohol, and engage in more promiscuous sex. A recent study in *Pediatrics* showed that even background television noise led to reduced attentiveness and learning in young children, and that the average child was getting four hours of background television noise each day. It is not just an association with television, but the absence of healthy activities that causes problems when the television is on: lack of social interaction, exercise, relaxation, and other fun activities that influence growth and development of young minds.

The National Institute of Mental Health reinforces the concerns of too much television viewing that spreads false health information from advertisements ("healthy" sugar cereal or "low-tar" cigarettes) as well as causing confusion for young children between reality and fantasy. One can only imagine this is more difficult now with the multitude of "reality" programs. More fear and confusion are the last things children need.

Now on to the commonsense part. When in doubt, turn the television off. Yes, it is easier to just give in and let kids watch whatever they want for as long as they want, but you are not doing anyone any favors long term. Television may seem like a lifesaver when you need a babysitter, but the downsides to television often outweigh the positives. If you are still looking for an out, use comedy shows judiciously as a coping technique or an intentional reward. They might help during a flare-up, as they distract attention from the pain while laughter releases endorphins. However, spending hours in front of the television on a regular basis disengages your child from real life. This stunts the young, plastic, developing brain.

Things you can do to have balanced television viewing:

- Arrange your household so that you can easily monitor your child's TV viewing.

- Choose quality programming.

- Put a time limit on TV.

- Allow TV after playing outside and finishing schoolwork or housework.

- Plan other laughter- and endorphin-stimulating activities each day to take the place of more television.

- Spend more face time together during the day without other distractions.

- Less is more. Shut it off and see what happens.

- At the very least, shut TV off during meals.

CHAPTER SUMMARY

- When we perceive something as stressful, our bodies react through our central nervous system, causing an increase in heart rate, blood pressure, breathing rate, stress hormones, and pain, and a disruption of the digestive rhythm.

- One way we can control our stress reaction is by practicing regular diaphragmatic breathing or visualization.

- Major adverse life events as well as chronic daily life stressors increase anxiety for children. Disruption or change at home affects children, whether or not we notice.

- Children with IBS are more likely to have anxiety or depression and are at higher risk for suicide. This needs to be evaluated and treated seriously.

- Assisting your child with the management of stress includes identifying thoughts and labeling emotions, as well as connecting these to physical sensations in the body.

- Routine is important for children to have an increased sense of control and to set their bodies in a comfortable cycle for optimal functioning.

- Small changes in your home can make a big difference, such as reducing time watching television and increasing time talking, preparing meals, or playing games as a family.

? QUESTIONS FOR YOUR FAMILY

Each family member can take a turn answering the following questions.

1) When do you feel the most stressed during the week?

2) When will you schedule time to truly relax and recover?

3) What will you do to relax and take care of yourself?

4) When do you feel best during the week? What are the circumstances?

5) How will you build on this optimal time to feel even better?

CHAPTER 6

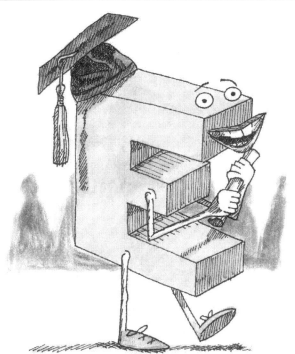

SEEDS: Education and Communication

To help your child successfully manage his IBS, you can learn to:

- Explain IBS to your child in understandable language.
- Listen carefully to understand your child's experience better.
- Ask your child and yourself the right questions.
- Support healthy behaviors by leading by example.
- Provide your child with adequate emotional support.

How Do I Explain IBS to My Child?

Depending on the age of your child, talking with him about anything might be like pulling teeth, and talking about his bowels might seem nearly impossible (with the exception of fart jokes). No matter what age, children are likely to be embarrassed, ashamed, and frustrated about what is happening.

For young children, simplify the explanation of IBS by locating and naming body parts. Describe what each organ does. Here is an example:

"Your tummy is one of the first stops that food makes as it goes from your mouth, down your esophagus, on the path all the way down through your intestines until you go to the bathroom. Your tummy works hard to use food for energy, to help you feel healthy, and pushes the rest through into the potty. When you feel nervous or scared about something, body parts inside get tired and scared, too, and do not work as well. Then your brain tells you that your tummy hurts."

In her *Treatment Manual for Recurrent Abdominal Pain,* Dr. Elizabeth Bigham suggests asking the child with IBS, "Who do you believe controls your tummy?" She emphasizes the importance of eliciting the beliefs that the child has, separate from what he may have been told by his parents or doctors. Dr. Bigham also suggests using analogies to help your child understand how his brain controls his tummy in a similar way that a coach tells members of the soccer team what to do, or a conductor tells the orchestra how to play. Each member of the team is important and tries her best to do a good job. When one member of the team is struggling, it is important to listen to what she (or the hurting body part) has to say. Let your child know the pain is real—although not dangerous—and is an important signal to pay attention to, because digestive symptoms are often a signal of stress.

> **Ask your child:** "If your tummy could talk, what would it say?" Children tell us so much if we are listening to what they are actually saying rather than what we think they should be saying. Listen without judgment and speak in a calm, loving, and matter-of-fact tone.

How Do I Talk to My Teenager about IBS?

Teenagers can handle a more sophisticated discussion about IBS. The key is to have open discussions where you are not bringing shame, accusations, or judgment to the problem. Explain as much as you have learned about IBS, from top to bottom (pun intended). One example might go like this:

"Our bodies have to work very hard to digest the food we eat into usable energy. Food travels down the esophagus to the stomach, through the small intestine, where much of it is absorbed, to the large intestine, and finally out the door. Sometimes this system does not function properly and can slow down, causing constipation, or speed up, causing diarrhea. Sometimes it does not even get that far, and you might feel tightness in your throat, an upset stomach, or even acid building and backpedalling up the esophagus.

"Stress is one main thing that can make IBS worse, and something we need to be aware of at home, at school, and with your friends. Your dad and I want to help you manage it better so you can enjoy more of the things you like to do. There are some relaxation and movement exercises in this book we would like to learn with you. Over time, we'll be trying new foods so you feel your best every day."

If your teen is now staring at you with a glazed-over look, don't give up. Stick with a clear, consistent, encouraging message to help him understand that the best treatment is a lifelong strategy of healthy coping habits (and lead by example the best you can).

Understanding Your Child's Experience

A difficult thing for many parents to fully comprehend is that children are not simply an extension of themselves, but rather completely separate human beings with an internal world all their own. Every child wants to feel heard and understood, necessary and loved. At the same time that children are trying to be recognized for being different, or individuating, they have a strong need to feel that they belong to a family as a valued member. This is a difficult balance.

chapter 6

Sara's mom started a routine of spending ten minutes with her each day just to check in. Not an interrogation, but just a present-moment "how are you?" Even if your teen looks at you like you are from Loserville at first, over time he will learn to trust you and use the opportunity however he needs to. What information he actually shares with you is not as important as simply spending the time to make a connection.

The Best Communication Tool: Listening

One of the best ways to support and communicate with your children is by listening. Not only will you learn more about them and their perspective, but listening builds trust. Here are some suggestions of how to practice this:

- Set aside some time to talk so you are not rushed.

- Really try to hear what they are sharing with you, not what you think they should be telling you.

- Spend time without talking, but simply doing something together, such as playing a game, washing dishes, or walking to the park.

- Use books and artwork as other ways for your children to relay important information to you that they cannot directly express.

- Listen at other unscheduled times—it may not be a scheduled sit-down discussion that reveals the most to you, but a chat in the car on the way to school, while packing lunches, or before falling asleep.

- Be open to listening to them at any time, even though you may not be solving the problem at that time.

- If the time is not good for you to talk, tell them you would like to hear more about it later, and be sure to do that.

- Do your best to make direct eye contact, crouching down to your child's height—if smaller than you—so it is less intimidating for him.

- Being put on the spot at dinner with "how was your day?" or "tell me about your friends" might increase stress at mealtime. Trying to force a conversation could backfire—being there is often enough.

- Avoid talking about your child to someone else in front of her as if she was not there. Include her in the conversation or keep it private.

- Build your child's trust by modeling how to keep private matters confidential (not gossiping), balanced with seeking information at the appropriate time and with the appropriate people—such as health care providers.

- Be patient. Healthy communication is a lifelong process that improves with practice.

- There may be other people your child wants to talk to about certain topics. Allow and encourage these healthy relationships.

Children understand a lot more than we think. They absorb adult words, behaviors, and emotions like sponges—even when they appear not to. But they lack the experience that allows them to have a broader adult perspective and make accurate interpretations. When parents have conflicts, children will often internalize the stress and present with abdominal complaints.

Exploring Your Child's Beliefs

Communicating with your child also includes asking the right questions. In a curious and supportive tone, ask her what she believes. The interrogation approach to "get to the bottom of this" will be counterproductive. Ask, "What do you think is going on with your tummy?" "What is most stressful to you at home?" This is an effort to understand what her beliefs are about herself and the situation from her point of view. Open-ended questions without judgment or correction leave room for a genuine response. The only goal is to understand more about what your child believes, not necessarily to change it.

Your only job at this point is to listen, listen, listen to what your child is telling you. It is not important that you agree; you are simply learning more about how she views the world. After she is done speaking, ask questions to clarify and make sure that you understand what she is saying. Nod and give other feedback when you think you understand. Then repeat back to her what you heard and ask if this is correct. Among all the opinions involved—yours, friends, family, the many physicians you may have consulted, television or Internet resources—your child's opinion is the most important. If she is mistaken, help her understand the truth.

Sara believed her parents loved her brother, Josh, more. Her parents acknowledged the truth of her feelings, but corrected the belief that she was loved less. They could understand how she felt that way, as Josh was older and had more privileges. But they reassured her that although life seemed unfair (indeed it is), their love for her was unwavering.

There can be lots of thoughts and beliefs that get in the way of understanding our children better.

Some beliefs that parents may have include:
- There is nothing wrong with my child.
- My child is not stressed.
- My child is very ill; something terrible is wrong with her.
- I try to make him talk, but he just won't talk to me, so I cannot fix it.
- He is going to become very sickly just like me (or someone else you know).
- He will never be normal.
- This is hopeless.
- He should not be so sensitive.
- If she would just do what I say, she would feel better.

Thoughts and beliefs that your child may have:
- I will never be able to go do the things I used to.
- I will always be in pain.
- No one cares about me.
- I should not be so sensitive.
- Someone should fix me.
- I will never be fixed.
- There is something terribly wrong with me that doctors cannot find.
- No one else has what I have.
- This is too embarrassing to talk about.
- I am alone in this.

Parenting Styles and Potential Traps

Having a child with IBS may be very stressful for you as a parent or caregiver. You may have already tried many different approaches to help your child and you're not sure what to do next. Whatever your general parenting style, it is important to neither be overly dramatic nor underplay the importance of your child's pain. Children look to their parents to see how strongly they should react to a situation. Remember that IBS is not imaginary, nor is it life threatening, and finding a balanced approach will help the entire family.

We are all trying to raise "successful" children, but what this means to each of us may be slightly different. Share your enthusiasm for life with your children through common interests. Teach them honesty, integrity, and creativity in daily tasks, large and small. A clean conscience brings better health, and creativity helps us manage stress and improve our problem-solving skills.

Everyone has different ways to parent, and each child has different needs. Depending on how we ourselves were raised, we are likely repeating our own past or overcompensating for it in some way. There are many ways to parent; however, extreme styles of overcoddling (enmeshed), permissive (detatched), controlling (authoritative), or chaotic (variable) parenting can exacerbate your child's symptoms and stunt his overall mental and emotional development.

Trap 1: Overly coddling and Enmeshed Parenting Style

An overcoddled child will likely display more illness behaviors because these are the behaviors that have been reinforced. If you are there to do everything for him, he is prevented from developing the necessary skills to function in everyday life. It sends the message that he cannot manage to become an independent, secure person. One sign of overly enmeshed parenting is if you are making all your child's day-to-day decisions or speaking for him frequently. You may notice you are chronically unhappy with his decisions and trying desperately to steer him in the "right" direction or the other extreme of believing your child can do no wrong. So-called "helicopter" parents hover over their child with the belief that they are protecting, but end up also hindering their development.

Trap 2: Permissive or Detached

Permissive parenting, on the other hand, also leads to insecurity and a lot of anxiety. Being allowed too much freedom leaves too much responsibility on children to regulate themselves and set their own limits. Secure children have consistent limits set for them and are clear what they are. Signs of being too detached include not *knowing* with whom your child spends time, what he watches on television, or what his favorites and interests are. Signs of being too permissive include not *caring* with whom your children spends time, what he watches on television, or what his favorites and interests are—or not setting age appropriate limits on the above.

Trap 3: Controlling or Authoritarian

Authoritarian parenting includes critical, controlling, and harsh behaviors often accompanied by rigid rules ("my way or the highway") and can also exacerbate IBS symptoms. An overcontrolled child may feel fearful of making a mistake or displeasing her parents and eventually feel a desperate need to break away from being micromanaged. (This does not preclude setting healthy limits.) A child feeling she can do no right will be fearful and frustrated. This can lead to depression, but at the very least decreases her sense of independence. At an unconscious level, asserting independence is more important to the development of a child than anything else. Your child wants to feel respected as a separate person, not like a parental appendage.

Trap 4: Chaotic

Sometimes, one parent is overreactive or dramatic and may overcoddle a sick child, while the other parent downplays or trivializes IBS. This inconsistent message is terribly confusing to children. One parent allows unlimited television while the other one restricts it until after homework; one allows unlimited snacks, the other restricts even healthy foods. Or perhaps, one parent changes his style depending on his mood—being too critical one moment, feeling guilty, and then being too permissive. The stress of chaotic messages can open the pain gate and send a mild tummy upset into a full-blown IBS flare-up. Don't worry if you suspect your child is trying to manipulate the situation with tummy aches. We

LAWSON & DEL POZO

all try to avoid things that make us feel bad especially if we lack the skills to cope with the situation. Rather than a lecture on being manipulative, children need support and new skills to navigate their day even when it seems disastrous.

School Options

Families often feel desperate and seek out educational alternatives. Some families may benefit from options that strike the right balance of structure for them. Private schools or homeschooling can help children thrive—as long as these options are enabling rather than disabling your child to manage life better. When faced with a big decision like changing schools, ask yourself if you are choosing it out of fear. If so, rethink it and see what makes good sense for your individual child in that particular situation. Most children can attend school as usual when home is a safe and steady place.

Coping

When it comes to coping, children have fewer resources than adults. They are dependent on their caregivers to teach them how to deal with life events. Children react naturally to whatever seems most likely to get their physical and emotional needs met. This may mean withdrawing, becoming combative and rebellious, becoming more ill, or finding other ways to influence their environment—and you are the primary source of their emotional and physical survival.

Children often tell themselves stories when they are unable to understand what is happening to them or around them (adults do, too). They believe these stories are true especially when they cannot comprehend an alternative explanation. They blame themselves if something is disrupted in the household—as commonly occurs with separation and divorce. By their very nature, children are egocentric and unable to have a broad understanding of complicated relationships. They cannot comprehend that family stress is not their fault.

Many children with IBS have a parent with IBS or anxiety. You, as their parent, may need to seek extra support to manage your symptoms and take back control of your life. Modeling how to ask and receive help

chapter 6

sets a powerful example. Set your household routine up for success to support everyone's needs and parent with confidence.

Boundaries and Assertiveness

Healthy boundaries make healthy, secure children. Assertive communication helps us set good boundaries with one another. Boundaries are simply boundaries, not rigid structures void of reason or discussion. Part of becoming a healthy and mature adult includes being able to communicate how we feel and what we want, directly and honestly, in a manner that is respectful to ourselves as well as other people. Assertive communication is neither defensive nor reactive. It is not hinting toward what we want, nor is it aggressive or mean-spirited.

> **Assertiveness is:** honest, respectful to self, respectful to others, clear, firm, based on love.
>
> **Assertiveness is not:** aggressive or mean-spirited, passively waiting for others to get the hint, defensive, reactive, or fear based.

You can speak assertively to your child when you want him to do something (clear, respectful, honest, and firm). Your child can learn to speak assertively to you, to siblings, to teachers, and to friends. Learning to say "no" and accept other people's "no" is an important part of maturing. This starts somewhere around age one, perhaps the dreaded "no! no! no!" from a toddler. It is an important word to learn as your child learns to pay attention to what her own needs are—and how to respect and take care of these needs. (Children gradually learn to self-soothe, just as they did when you let them cry in the crib for the first time.)

An overcontrolling parent enforces his own "no," but does not respect the child's "no." An overly permissive parenting style caters to the child's "no" but does not teach the child to respect other people's "no." Either way, a child who does not learn healthy boundaries early on may struggle with problems later—such as saying no to drugs and alcohol, limiting food proportions, managing money, or navigating other risk situations.

Children need to learn to give and take boundaries (noes) in a healthy way. Respecting each other's "noes" does not mean giving in. It does mean listening to each other and allowing disagreement in the household. It is OK if you and your son disagree about what "violent television" is. Allow your child to have different opinions from you; in fact, encourage it. Allow discussions to understand his perspectives better and help you stay in touch with what he is experiencing at school or home. Your answer to watching certain movies might remain "no," depending on the content and the age of your child, but you will get to know him as a separate person with preferences, tastes, opinions, and ideas. The connection between you remains intact and likely strengthens.

Your child's age will determine how you go about enforcing boundaries and allowing natural consequences. You would not allow your four-year-old to find out for herself that not wearing mittens can lead to frostbite. You can say that you understand she does not like wearing mittens, but that in order to go sledding she must put them on.

As your children become teens, they get better at making choices on their own. You have been nudging them toward adulthood with support. Even with a teen, setting healthy boundaries doesn't need to involve yelling or door slamming (on your part, at least). A good sign that you have been setting healthy limits all along is that you do not reach the boiling point. Stephany lied and skipped class, leading to the natural consequence of her dad, John, having to drive her to school instead of allowing her the freedom to drive. Stephany was angry about this, and John acknowledged her feelings and stuck to his decision despite the additional inconvenience for him. Once Stephany was attending class and her grades were up, the terms could be renegotiated.

At each age, remember it is natural for children to test the boundaries you set. This is no excuse for bad behavior—think of it as their job. And your job, although exhausting, is to keep setting limits to help them grow up to be responsible adults who can set limits with themselves and others. We do this for them from the time they are dependent on us, and less and less as we prepare to release them from the nest. Adolescence is not the time to crack down and control them more, but to continue to give good structure and make informed decisions. Let them figure out things for themselves on choices with safe outcomes either way (although perhaps not ideal). You wouldn't say to your sixteen-year-old, "Well, Tom, it is your choice to drink and drive." That is not safe or within reason. However, if Tom wants to stay up late, you might say, "It is up to you to get to bed on time tonight so you are not tired tomorrow." You wouldn't have this same response for a preschooler about bedtime. But as children grow into each developmental stage, you allow them more freedoms that naturally bring more responsibility.

Once a child has the skills to communicate assertively, help him cope with how the situation might play out. The answer may still be "no," but assertive communication (clear, respectful, honest, and firm) leaves room for negotiation. It reduces misunderstandings and gives all parties a chance to be heard before a decision is reached.

Sara learned to set boundaries with her brother by asking Josh to please leave her room when she felt irritated with him. This reduced arguments between them, and she was better equipped to say "no" to peer pressure at school. She felt more confident asking her teacher to allow her to sit in the back of the classroom so it would not be so obvious when she needed to go to the bathroom. Previously, she could not talk about it or look her teacher in the eye. Years later, when she asked for a car, the answer was still no, but her parents heard her out and understood it was a sense of freedom that she really desired. They were able to accommodate her in other ways that supported her independence.

CHAPTER SUMMARY

- Explain IBS to your children in understandable language, listening with empathy to what they already believe about their bodies.

- It is important for you to know their symptoms are real, a useful clue that they are stressed, but not dangerous or life-threatening.

- All children have a natural need to individuate, or a desire to be recognized for who they are. Their deepest aspiration is for you to "get" them.

- Common traps parents can fall into include overreacting to symptoms with rewards or coddling, or reacting with criticism or dismissiveness. Permissive and chaotic parenting styles can also increase stress.

- Setting healthy, loving, consistent boundaries is difficult, but necessary to build strong relationships.

- Good communication skills will help children manage stress and minimize symptoms and will assist them in relationships the rest of their lives.

? QUESTIONS FOR YOUR FAMILY

Each family member can take a turn answering the following questions.

1) When will you take time each week to listen to one another?

2) What signal will you share to let each other know when you need a break?

3) What will you change in your home environment to support listening to each other and communicating better?

CHAPTER 7

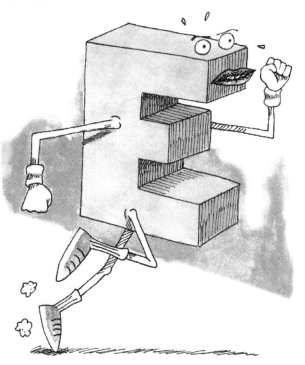

SEEDS: Exercise with All Fours

Exercise is the second E in SEEDS, a vital component of our program for the management of IBS; but we are not going to give you another lecture on exercise or write a dissertation on all the health benefits of it. It's pretty simple; daily movement is a necessary good and can be rewarding if paired with a fun activity. We need to move our bodies to feel good—think arms and legs, or "all fours." In studies of college students, collegiate athletes suffered less from IBS than their inactive college counterparts. One study even showed a "dose response," meaning that those who exercised vigorously did better than students who exercised moderately. The group that exercised moderately, in turn, did better than those who did not exercise at all.

Following are four reasons to exercise for IBS, four types of exercises, and four examples of each.

Four Reasons to Exercise

1) **Exercise reduces IBS pain:** A few controlled research trials have revealed significant improvement in many IBS symptoms with exercise. Exercise may reduce pain by increasing the production of endorphins, pleasure chemicals that circulate around the brain in the cerebrospinal fluid. Exercise closes the pain gate and reduces visceral hypersensitivity. Drug companies realize the role of endorphins in blocking pain pathways and are continually designing drugs that look and act just like endorphins. It is safer and cheaper to utilize our brain's natural ability to create endorphins, rather than take pills.

2) **Exercise improves intestinal motility:** Exercise improves the ability of the gut to move food through expeditiously by way of the vagus nerve. The vagus nerve helps the stomach to accommodate food and empty effectively.

3) **Exercise improves overall health and well-being, reduces stress, and increases happiness:** Exercise helps your central nervous system work more efficiently and induces a natural relaxation response. Feel-good chemicals such as serotonin and dopamine are released during exercise and help us sleep deeply, regulate appetite, and elevate mood. A recent study from Sweden showed moderate exercise for thirty minutes five times a week resulted in a significant improvement of IBS symptoms and general quality of life. On top of that, a sense of well-being, sleep, energy, and social interactions all improved. However, anxiety and depression scores as well as stool patterns remained unchanged, emphasizing, as we have found, that exercise alone cannot treat IBS.

4) **Exercise helps maintain a healthy weight:** People who are obese are 2.6 times more likely to have IBS than nonobese people. Processing large amounts of food can trigger pain, bloating, or constipation. Emotional overeating can trigger problems because the gut is both stressed and taxed with excess food. In addition, instilling good exercise habits into a child's life will set him up for success the rest of his life. Children will be more likely to keep exercise as a daily habit, like most habits, when they learn it early on.

Four Ways to get Adequate Movement

1) **Stability ball and tubing exercises:** for balance, coordination, and strength.

2) **Cardiovascular activity:** to increase circulation and relaxation response.

3) **Yoga, breathing, and stretching:** for flexibility, strength, and sense of well-being.

4) **Daily routine:** doing what you love, playing, and integrating movement into daily habits.

1) Stability ball and tubing

Bob, the physical trainer we work with in our SEEDS program, teaches simple and fun exercises using stability balls and cable tubing. The focus is on core strengthening, starting with four-point balance (on hands and knees). The exercises can easily be practiced at home. This practical approach helps the children see past the "I can'ts." Since movement is cumulative, children can spend several minutes exercising when they feel the need to blow off steam or take a break from homework. Exercise energizes them and helps them refocus. When gas accumulates in our intestines, the natural response is to tighten our abdominal wall muscles. The opposite tends to happen in IBSers, resulting in the uncomfortable sensation of bloating. Intuitively, it would seem that increasing abdominal muscle tone could minimize subsequent bloating; simply sitting on the stability ball while doing homework has a positive effect on core muscles and improves overall posture and back support.

chapter 7

FOUR STABILITY BALL EXERCISES

   a.   Four-point balance

   b.   Sitting position

   c.   Roll out

   d.   Supine floor bridge

FOUR TUBING EXERCISES (EXERCISE BAND)

   a.   Squats

   b.   Standing row

   c.   Chest press

   d.   Alternating row

> Checkout **thegutsolution.com** for additional exercises you can add to your daily routine!

GENERAL GUIDELINES:

- Practice every other day or three times per week.
- Do twelve to twenty repetitions of each.
- Do two to four circuits of all the exercises.
- Work as hard as you can on each exercise.
- Eat healthy foods to support your workouts.
- Relax after your workouts.

2) Cardiovascular movement

Cardiovascular exercise is achieved when arms and legs are moving rhythmically to increase heart rate. This does not mean that children should pound a treadmill. They shouldn't! They shouldn't pump iron or anything else that will lead them to hate exercising. Children should play. Remember that? Gathering a group of neighbor children together for a game of kickball or tag all afternoon until you were forced back into the house by your parents calling you for dinner? In our highly technological age, it takes more effort to stay active. It might be easier to allow your child to stay plugged into electronics, but the down side may be an exacerbation of IBS symptoms.

FOUR EXAMPLES OF CARDIOVASCULAR ACTIVITY

a. Skipping rope (teach your children the old jump rope rhymes)

b. Running games outside with other children: soccer, basketball, kickball, tag

c. Martial arts

d. Swimming, walking, jogging

3) Yoga

Yoga embraces both physicality and relaxation. SEEDS introduces yoga as a prelude to guided imagery for relaxation. A pilot study in the Netherlands in 2012 showed reduced pain and frequency of bowel problems for IBSers who practiced yoga. Another study showed that two months of yoga resulted in a significant decrease in bowel symptoms and anxiety—compared to conventional treatment—by enhancing parasympathetic nervous system reactivity (the relaxation response) as measured by heart rate parameters (heart rate variability). The University of California, Los Angeles, recently introduced yoga into their pediatric pain management program.

The word yoga means union of mind and body. The ancient science of yoga has been practiced in the East for thousands of years, bringing health, happiness, and improved quality of life. Practiced gently and regularly, the postures will also increase levels of fitness and flexibility. (Although yoga came from ancient religious practices, the West has adapted it as a separate movement practice from religious worship.)

Breathing sequences are a key part of yoga that enhance parasympathetic output—the healing and relaxing side of your nervous system (see chapter 5). Breathe in diaphragmatically as the body stretches and expands; breathe out as the body contracts or folds forward. Different poses strengthen the lungs and tone various structures, including the spine. Hold each pose for ten seconds to a minute.

chapter 7

YOGA POSES:

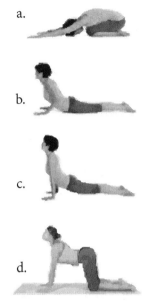

a. Child's pose

b. Cobra

c. Up-Dog

d. Cow

4) Be active in daily life

Integrate movement into your family's culture by walking to places when you can. Walk or bike to the library, store, or park on a regular basis. Take the stairs or park at the opposite end of the parking lot. Rake your own leaves (and then enjoy jumping into them). Dr. Lawson can be seen biking to work rain or shine. He practices martial arts with friends each weekend, and he and Helen walk their dog, Niko, twice a day. Dr. Del Pozo bikes her daughter to school twice a week and walks to the grocery store, hauling food back in the stroller. It's time spent with her daughter, too. Keep movement fun and build it in to become part of your family's weekly routine. Suggestions for daily movement:

a. Walk to school whenever possible (safe, good weather), and walk the dog.

b. Help with yard work or other house projects.

c. Park far away from store or walk to store with wagon.

d. Bike to the library, park, or school.

In general, we emphasize noncompetetive exercises at SEEDS since the last thing we want to do to children with IBS is to introduce more stress. The exercise routine we teach is semistructured to give children movement skills to use in a nonrigid way.

Although more exercise is likely to help your child manage IBS better and have a better quality of life, extreme exercise along with anxiety can cancel out the benefits. Extreme exercise can result in more fluid secretion into the intestinal lumen (where nutrients are absorbed). Some high-endurance athletes, particularly rowers, cyclists, and runners, have a higher prevalence of lower GI symptoms such as bloating, cramping, and diarrhea. We have seen quite a few highly competitive athletes in SEEDS. The imposed need to win results in greater mental stress, which produces more bowel symptoms. A recent study showed that college rowers have more IBS symptoms than their inactive college counterparts. Although this seems to contradict that exercise helps manage IBS, it may be that demanding schedules, high-endurance exercise, early-morning starts, and highly competitive elements reduce the advantages that exercise alone provides. We all want our children to succeed, but too much pressure along with extreme exercise can be harmful.

CHAPTER SUMMARY

- Exercise can reduce IBS pain, increase gut motility, reduce stress, improve one's general sense of well-being, and help maintain a healthy weight.

- Core muscle tone can be achieved through practicing stability ball and tubing exercises.

- Cardiovascular exercise relieves stress and improves the relaxation response and overall conditioning and fitness.

- Yoga increases core strength, flexibility, and quality of life.

- Integrate movement into your lives as a regular part of each day. Be creative, play ball, walk, or bike somewhere together, and have fun.

chapter 7

？ QUESTIONS FOR YOUR FAMILY

Each family member can take a turn answering the following questions.

1) What games or other activities do you find to be the most fun?

2) When will you take time to move throughout the day?

3) What will you do and with whom?

CHAPTER 8

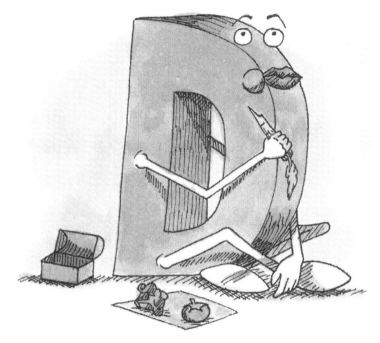

SEEDS: Diet – How and What to Eat

Menus and advice from Monica Randel, Registered Dietitian

> " *T*he secret to feeding a healthy family is to love good food, trust yourself, and share that love and trust with your child. When the joy goes out of eating, nutrition suffers." - Ellyn Satter

In this chapter, we will:

- Provide general nutritional guidelines
- Discuss behaviors to mitigate the intensity of flare-ups
- Suggest foods to manage specific symptoms

Gas, bloating, constipation, and diarrhea—it all sounds like a dietary problem, but it isn't. As hard as that may be to believe, food is not the cause of IBS. Millions of diet books are sold each year promising to "cure" digestive problems; and although many people find relief with diet changes, food is not the cause of the problem. However, most people feel better when they eat better, and certain foods can certainly make IBS symptoms worse. So, yes, eat healthier, but don't drive yourselves or each other crazy doing it.

More importantly, consider the environment the food is going into— the sensitive, irritable gut and its low tolerance for stress from challenging foods and from emotions. Stressful emotions set up the gut to feel that food is the enemy. Depending on the environment, food can feel like an intruder rather than something good for us. A peanut butter and jelly sandwich may feel fine one day but terrible the next. The food might remain the same, but the conditions of the environment it entered changed.

A bad diet can surely flare IBS symptoms, just as a good diet can help turn it down a notch. Overall, eating a variety of wholesome foods over a life span is best. This advice does not seem to change despite food fads. We'll get to more food details after first discussing that how you eat is just as or more important than what you eat.

How You Eat Matters

Eating behavior impacts the amount of pain and bloating your child experiences, as well as daily energy levels and the mind's ability to concentrate. A common pattern for children with IBS is to skip breakfast because their tummies hurt, eat little or no lunch (feeling anxious about what symptoms it will trigger), then feel so hungry in the afternoon that they chow down whatever food is readily available as quickly as possible. This adds to the vicious cycle of feeling sick, avoiding food, poor eating choices, and gulping air with chunks of food while eating too fast. A fear and avoidance cycle with food is common in IBS. But avoiding food is not the answer; following good eating habits is definitely part of the solution.

Healthy Eating Behaviors:

- Relax while eating: Avoid multitasking, sit down, take your time, and arrange the environment around you to be clutter free and peaceful.

- Practice mindful eating: Savor each bite. Smell, taste, and feel the texture.

- Eat small meals: Eating large quantities can stretch the capacity of the stomach, sending unhappy messages to and from the brain.

- Chew food slowly: Eating slowly and chewing your foods carefully can help the stomach have an easier time moving food along.

- Chew each bite well: Practice chewing your food at least twenty times before swallowing.

- Take breaks between bites to avoid eating too fast and swallowing air.

- Allow plenty of time to digest after eating: Rest for fifteen minutes before getting up or going for an easy walk.

Dietician and psychotherapist Ellyn Satter emphasizes having a healthy relationship with food, developing trust in yourself and in food, and building that relationship with your child. Despite good intentions, it does not work to force-feed children or be very restrictive with food. Arguing, coaxing, rewarding, and punishing are all approaches that will set up mistrust in the relationship. Eating should be an easygoing and pleasurable experience, not an opportunity to either be "good" or "bad."

> **Division of responsibility:** the responsibility of the parent to provide healthy food options—what is to be eaten, when, and where. The child is responsible for what she chooses from the options on the table, how much she eats, and also whether she eats at all.

Satter uses the term *division of responsibility,* referring to the responsibility of the parent to provide healthy food options—what is to be eaten, when, and where. The child is responsible for what she chooses from the options on the table, how much she eats, and also whether she eats at all. This requires parents to plan ahead, making a balanced and sustainable meal plan for the family. A casual approach is best, removing all tension

chapter 8

and criticism from the food relationship. Parents need to trust their children will eat enough of what they need and also trust themselves not to give in to old habits that create tension around mealtime. Children learn from parents how to relate to food and make the best choices for themselves as they mature.

What is a Balanced Diet?

A balanced meal is one that combines adequate energy, protein, and nutrients that our bodies need for the next four hours. Every time you eat, try to get a portion of carbohydrates to keep up good energy and concentration. This means *complex carbohydrates* like brown rice or quinoa, not simple carbs like cookies and chips. Protein is needed for building and repairing and is commonly found in lean meats and fish and, to a lesser degree, in whole grains. Fruits and vegetables provide the *antioxidants, vitamins,* and *phytochemicals* to protect and heal our bodies. Fat usually comes along for the ride in protein or carbohydrate foods, and we do not need to go out of our way to find more of it. But the type of fat does matter. Plant-based fats (like avocados, olive oil, or nuts) and some fish oils are optimal because they trigger less inflammation and are healthier to digest than animal fats. Good fats help our brains work properly and also tell us we feel full after a meal.

We have heard so many times during our lives that "we are what we eat." This has become a cliché because it is true! A solid food foundation will give us a better chance of achieving our full potential as healthy humans. Eating a variety of fresh foods is key. Variety provides different antioxidants and phytochemicals that keep us healthy for the long haul. Rather than prescribe a rigid diet, move toward what we like to call "intelligent flexibility." This means using the best information available and your common sense. Rules of thumb:

- Eat a variety of whole foods.
- Eat at regular intervals (three or four meals per day).
- Avoiding highly processed, sugary, and fatty foods.

We all make decisions each day at each meal about how to take care of ourselves as far as what we put into our bodies. Eating healthy does not have to be an "extreme makeover" version; however, some children in SEEDS felt relief within just one week of avoiding trigger foods (like pepperoni pizza or milkshakes). Do the best you can to put out the best food available to feed your family.

The stomach is one of the first places for food to stop on the journey of digestion. If a food is too fatty or sugary, the stomach may rebel and cause the rest of the intestinal tract to react. In general, a low-fat and low-sugar diet can be a great place to start. You guessed it, this means trading cake, ice cream, cookies, sodas, cheeseburgers, and other highly processed foods for more wholesome foods. (We are sorry if that made you groan, but ask yourself how badly you want to feel better.) Some people with IBS also find that they cannot handle lactose well. There are many nondairy milk alternatives, such as soy, rice, or almond milk.

Eating for Symptom Management

Typically, our body is amazingly adaptive to different diets, but the IBS gut is not as tolerant. Nutrition for an IBSer can be altered in order to manage diarrhea, bloating, constipation, and/or stomach pain. Depending on your symptoms, you can help alleviate some of your body's reaction by choosing foods that are easier for your gut to handle. It can be very frustrating to read all the dietary recommendations for IBS, especially when some appear to contradict each other. But hang in there. Since the symptoms of IBS can change daily, your diet may need to also change frequently to adapt. If your child has more than one symptom at a time, you might fret about which diet to follow. Multiple symptoms are not uncommon. Remember these rules of thumb:

- Follow your instincts: go with the diet recommendation to reduce the worst symptom at the time.
- Try the recommendations that sound right for you and your child's individual gut.
- There is no one-size-fits-all diet, and menus may need to be modified for the individual.
- Make changes slowly. Do not try too many things at once or you will not be able to figure out what is helping or what is hurting.

chapter 8

Staying on a preventative diet when you feel better will not necessarily prevent a flare-up. (Remember, it is not the food's fault.) As soon as you are feeling better, reintegrate small amounts of the foods you are used to eating back into your diet. The goal is to become comfortable with food. Remember, what we eat is just a part of the puzzle for the complicated picture of IBS, and by working on stress management, exercise, relaxation, and sleep, you should be able to enjoy a good variety of healthy foods.

Identifying Common Food Triggers

Identifying trigger foods may seem like a monumental task. Below are some of the most common ingredients to avoid—especially during an IBS flare. While we might think we know what constitutes a good diet, what is fine for a normal digestive system may be wrong for a child with IBS. And what helps a child suffering from constipation may utterly undo a child who struggles with excessive gas. To add to the confusion, many children with IBS contend with gas, bloating, constipation, diarrhea, stomach pain, and acid reflux in an ongoing hellish rotation. Solving one symptom with a dietary fix may trigger another.

What to Eat and Avoid for Relief from Gas and Bloating

Gas comes from the bacteria fermentation of undigested food; in other words, from the byproducts of digested fiber. Although this is a good thing, it can cause excessive gas. Everyone has a different intestinal bacteria makeup in her gut, which explains why some people have more vocal bowels than others. Gas can also be from swallowing too much air while eating. If your child is gassy, the goal is to minimize the air and bacterial gas production in the intestinal tract. Start by practicing these behaviors:

- Chew with your mouth closed.
- Do not drink through a straw.
- Do not talk while eating.
- No bubbles (sodas, bubbly water).
- Avoid gas-forming foods such as beans and lentils.

- Avoid chewing gum.
- Eat slowly.

The **FODMAP** (Fermentable, Oligo-, Di-, and Monosaccharides and Polyols) diet can help prevent the bacteria in our gut from making excessive gas. There is no need to completely eliminate these foods, but it is important not to provide too much fuel for the bacteria at one time. This is one time where a food diary can help. If there is a pattern of more gas production with some of the foods on the list, then your family can reduce the intake of that food. To say it again: reduce these foods, but do not necessarily exclude them altogether.

Avoiding sugary foods will help reduce gas and may also improve energy and concentration. Sugars come in different forms with many names, so avoiding them can be tricky. You want to limit foods with excess fructose, fructans, sorbitol, and raffinose. You have to read the ingredients carefully to recognize these. Once you get the hang of it, it will become easier. These are four types of sugars to watch for.

1. Fructose (corn syrup, sodas)

The single biggest offender of the fructose category is high fructose corn syrup. High fructose corn syrup makes up most sodas and many cookies and other snacks. Even some healthy foods are high in fructose and can also make an IBS flare-up worse. These include fruit juices, coconut milk and coconut cream, and honey. Skip the fruit juices or reduce to one-third cup, or dilute the juice with water to minimize gas and bloating. Many fruits are also high in fructose and may need to be eaten in moderation. These include apples, pears, mandarins, mango, watermelon, honeydew melon, nashi, carambola or star fruit, and peaches. Even one tablespoon of dried fruit can have a lot of fructose; however, sugary snacks and sodas have the most fructose with the least nutritional value.

2. Fructans

You will also want to limit sugars in the fructan category for bloating and gas. This includes foods that have large amounts of wheat and rye, including many breads and other baked goods. Limit onions of many types (brown, white, spring, Spanish, shallots, leeks), artichokes, zucchini, and chicory that is found in Ecco and Caro drinks. Inulin is an artificial fiber added to products like dairy foods and snack bars. Fructo-oligo saccharides (FOS) are an artificial fiber added to some nutritional supplements to be aware of.

3. Sorbitol

Sorbitol is often added to diet foods as a sugar substitute. However, it is a laxative and can increase gastrointestinal distress with gas or diarrhea. (It may also be why prunes do what they do.) You can recognize foods containing sorbitol by reading ingredients of artificial sweeteners like sorbitol, mannitol, xylitol, and isomalt. Watch out for any artificially sweetened gums, mints, or candy. Fruits that are high in sorbitol include apricots, peaches, nectarines, cherries, plums, apples, and pears, so eat these in moderation and avoid them during a flare-up.

4. Raffinose

Raffinose is called a trisaccharide, which means it is made of glactose, fructose, and glucose. To reduce gas and bloating, limit these high-raffinose foods: cabbage, brussels sprouts, green beans, asparagus, and legumes like chickpeas, lentils, red kidney beans, and baked beans. The amount eaten at one time seems to determine how uncomfortable a child may feel. You could try eating these foods in small portions, taking a break, and eating another small portion later.

Menu Examples

Menus for the patient with IBS with gas and bloating (FODMAP DIET):

	Day One	Day Two	Day Three
Breakfast	» rice cereal with lactose-free milk » banana » egg	» oatmeal with blueberries and nuts » drizzle of maple syrup » lactose-free milk	» Greek yogurt with strawberries and sugar » rice cake with peanut butter
Snack	» rice crackers	» orange	» tangelo
Lunch	» turkey, tuna, or peanut butter sandwich on gluten-free bread, small amount of mayonnaise » baked potato chips » mandarin orange	» chicken or beef tacos on corn tortilla with cheddar cheese, lettuce, and tomato	» chicken and rice soup with rice crackers

Snack	» low-fat popcorn	» cantaloupe	» corn tortilla chips with a little hard cheese (such as cheddar) melted on top
Dinner	» lean cooked beef, fish, pork, chicken, or turkey » baked potato with pat of butter » carrots	» lean cooked beef, fish, pork, chicken, or turkey » rice or quinoa pasta » green beans	» lean cooked beef, fish, pork, chicken, or turkey » quinoa » corn

What to Eat to Manage Diarrhea

The first step to managing diarrhea dietarily is to replace electrolytes from lost fluids. However, many people choose fluids that can make diarrhea worse. Drinks often contain high fructose corn syrup (energy drinks, sports drinks, sodas) that can make the gut move faster and increase diarrhea. It is a much better idea to use one of the pediatric formulas and water it down, or make your own sports drink. Here are two low-sugar options that will still replenish electrolytes.

Sports Drink Recipe

1 quart water

1 teaspoon salt

4 teaspoons sugar

1 heaping teaspoon baking soda.

Boil 3–5 minutes. Refrigerate. You can flavor with lemon, lime, or fruit juice.

Fluid Replacement Recipe

1 cup orange juice (substitute a noncitrus juice, such as pear nectar, if mouth sores are present; avoid grape juice, which can worsen diarrhea)

8 teaspoons sugar

3/4 teaspoon baking soda

1/2 teaspoon salt

1 quart (4 cups) water

BRATT Diet: Bananas, Rice, Tea, Toast

This diet is soft, easy to digest, low acid, low fat, low gastric irritant, and low fiber. Besides the BRATT diet, here are some other foods choices with ingredients that won't exacerbate diarrhea.

Foods to manage diarrhea include:

- Plainly cooked, soft-textured, low-fat proteins (braised, boiled or poached fish, chicken or turkey)
- Scrambled or poached eggs prepared without fat
- Tofu
- Low-fat cheese and cottage cheese
- Cooked soft vegetables—avoid the legumes
- Peeled, cooked, or canned fruits (in their own juices rather than sugar)
- Broths and low-fat soups without beans
- Diluted fruit juices
- Rice milk
- Unsweetened nonbran cold and hot cereals
- Breads without seeds and nuts, as long as they are not high in bran/fiber
- White or egg noodles (served plain or in broth)
- White rice (served plain or in broth)
- Quinoa (served plain or in broth)
- White couscous (served plain or in broth)
- White part of the potato (baked or boiled)
- Peeled yam or sweet potato
- Flour tortilla
- Low-fiber crackers
- Rice cakes

Menus for Diarrhea

	Day One	Day Two	Day Three
Breakfast	» Cream of Rice cereal » applesauce » diluted apple or cranberry juice	» low-fat cottage cheese » fruit, toast	» eggs » toast, easy on the butter » weak tea
Snack	» canned pears	» vanilla wafers	» canned peaches
Lunch	» turkey or tuna on bread, small amount of mayonnaise » rice milk	» chicken and rice soup » saltine crackers » vanilla pudding » weak tea	» flour tortilla, low-fat cheese quesadilla » chicken or vegetable broth
Snack	» fruit popsicle	» low-fat yogurt	» graham crackers
Dinner	» lean cooked beef, fish, pork, chicken, or turkey » baked potato with pat of butter » well-cooked carrots	» lean cooked beef, fish, pork, chicken, or turkey » couscous or rice » well-cooked green beans	» lean cooked beef, fish, pork, chicken, or turkey » quinoa » cooked zucchini

Foods to Manage Constipation

You may already know what to eat for constipation: fiber! Preventing constipation is easier than treating it once children are backed up. Once a person is constipated, fiber simply makes the stool behind the problem area softer.

There are two types of fiber: insoluble and soluble. Insoluble fiber tends to help us stay more regular because it does not get as soft as soluble fiber. It pushes on the colon to send the message to the brain to move things along. To prevent constipation, try eating foods higher in insoluble fiber, such as these:

- Bran: bran muffins, bran flakes, and other high fiber cereals
- Whole grains, vegetables, and fruits with skin
- Nuts

Remember to increase fiber slowly. About half of the people in one study felt more bloated and gassy with high fiber diets.

Soluble fiber increases the bacterial content of stool. Bacteria are 95 percent water; therefore, soluble fiber bulks the stool by holding in more water. There are a lot of products out there now that add fiber to regular products, such as crackers, breads, breakfast bars, and tortillas. Read food labels to find products that have this added fiber. The best sources for soluble fiber are:

- oatmeal

- beans

- legumes

- fruit

Prunes, or dried plums, also help our colons move along. There is a special ingredient in prunes that stimulates the colon. Snack on prunes or cut them up and add them to other snacks or cereal.

A discussion of constipation would not be complete without a reminder to drink enough fluid, get plenty of physical activity, and make time to use the bathroom on a regular basis.

Menus for Constipation

	Day One	Day Two	Day Three
Breakfast	» high fiber cereal » almond milk » strawberries or raspberries	» oatmeal with added ground flaxseed, blueberries and nuts	» eggs » high fiber toast » grapefruit
Snack	» high fiber crackers	» orange	» high fiber granola bar
Lunch	» turkey, tuna, or peanut butter sandwich, high fiber bread, small amount of mayonnaise » apple with peel	» chicken or beef burrito on corn tortilla with beans, small amount of cheddar cheese, lettuce and tomato	» lentil or bean soup with whole grain crackers
Snack	» trail mix with nuts and dried fruit	» cut-up cucumber, carrot, and celery with small amount of low-fat dressing	» corn tortilla chips » with mild salsa
Dinner	» lean cooked beef, fish, pork, chicken, or turkey » baked sweet potato with pat of butter » carrots	» lean cooked beef, fish, pork, chicken, or turkey » whole grain pasta » green beans	» lean cooked beef, fish, pork, chicken, or turkey » quinoa » salad with fresh vegetables

What to Eat and Avoid for Indigestion or Dyspepsia

There are many terms for functional dyspepsia: acid indigestion, reflux, acidy stomach, or gastroesophogeal reflux disorder (GERD). High fat and highly acidic foods distend the stomach and delay emptying of it, leading to reflux and/or bloating. For indigestion eat leaner proteins (such as chicken breast or tuna) and avoid these foods:

- Caffeine in coffee, sodas, tea, or chocolate
- Fatty, greasy foods such as burgers, hot dogs, and pizza
- Acidy foods such as orange and grapefruit, tomato, kiwi, pineapple
- Pepper
- Peppermint (for some people)
- Bell peppers and hot peppers
- Alcohol

What to do:
- Eat smaller meals.
- Eat more frequent meals.
- Drink enough water, but not too much during a meal.

What Should I Do for Stomach Pain?

Stomach pain is more challenging to manage with diet and responds to stress management and exercise much better. Most physicians and dietitians will suggest clear liquids until the pain passes. Clear liquids include:
- water
- weak tea
- watered-down apple juice
- broth

Less food is generally better when your stomach hurts. Fluids are crucial so that you do not get dehydrated. Ice chips and popsicles may work best because the rate of the liquid hitting the stomach is slow. Then, as the pain lessens, increase the diet to a bland diet, such as the one in the diarrhea section. Also, use relaxation techniques from chapter 5 to reduce tension in the stomach muscles that are tightening and guarding around the pain.

Some people have found they had fewer tummy aches using ginger-based products such as raw ginger, ginger snaps, ginger tea, and candied ginger. Other research says that peppermint oil may help, although not much better than a placebo. If you want to try peppermint, take an enteric-coated preparation to avoid the sensation of heartburn and rectal burning.

Managing Nausea

Many children complain of nausea, especially in the morning after trying to eat breakfast. It may be less about the food than the rush we are in to eat it in anticipation of the day! We need to provide enough time to chew our food well so the stomach can accommodate it at an easy pace. Strong odors may increase reactivity to foods; therefore, eat cold foods that are not as odorous as hot foods. Try cold cereals that are low in sugar and fairly easy to digest. You can even let it get a little mushy or try:

- smoothies
- cottage cheese
- yogurt
- soft cereals: Cream of Wheat, oatmeal, or any cooked and cooled whole grain

It can be confusing and even frustrating to have more than one intestinal issue at one time: some diarrhea, then constipation, pain, gas, and bloating. Other times symptoms come and go and the diets seem so different you might not know which one to follow. When in doubt, err on the side of caution. You can treat several problems together. For example, Sara is having gas and constipation. She considered eating beans for increased fiber, but realized that is not a good idea because beans are on the avoid list for gas. She decided to go with sweet potatoes, a safer fiber choice.

These lists can guide you; however, a dietitian can help tailor your diet to include all the necessary nutrients and individualize it to fit your lifestyle.

CHAPTER SUMMARY

- Eat a variety of nutritious, whole, unprocessed foods without completely eliminating any one category without good reason.

- How we eat is more important than what we eat. Eat sitting down in a relaxed environment. Chew food well, eat slowly, and savor it.

- Nurture a healthy relationship with food by eating according to symptoms, but do not obsess about food or avoid it like the enemy. More stress about food will make symptoms worse.

- Limit high sugar (especially high fructose corn syrup) and fatty foods—especially during a flare-up.

- See the suggested menus to get a feel for what to eat for the current IBS symptom your child is experiencing.

❓ QUESTIONS FOR YOUR FAMILY

Each family member can take a turn answering the following questions. Feel free to write in the spaces below.

- What will we change around the table to make the eating experience more enjoyable?

- What food triggers have you already identified? What will you substitute for this food (especially during a flare-up?)

- What is your favorite whole (unpackaged) food?

- Fill in the blanks: "I feel good when I eat more _____ _____ and less _____."

CHAPTER 9

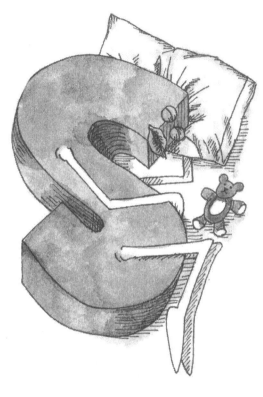

SEED⑤: Sleep

The Importance of Sleep

Insomnia is often one of a cluster of symptoms that can occur with IBS. At least 15 percent of children are not getting enough sleep—for various reasons. Not scheduling enough time to sleep is a different problem than feeling too restless or anxious to fall or stay asleep. Many people with IBS have trouble fully relaxing and sleeping deeply. We've all had disrupted sleep from simply staying up too late having fun, but for some children sleep is easily disrupted with any amount of change or stress. Some children fear bedtime because they often wake up with stomach pain.

Without good quality (delta-wave) sleep, even healthy people end up having body aches and pain, poor concentration, and changes in mood, and are more likely to become overweight or obese. Adults who work night-shift and especially swing-shift are more likely to suffer from IBS than day-shift workers. We need good quality sleep to allow us to feel good and have enough energy to do the activities we want to do. Sleep

117

helps our cells repair, encodes memories, conserves our body's resources, reduces stress hormones, and increases endorphins (natural painkilling chemicals). However, nighttime is a prime time for worries and fears to make themselves known. Stress can easily disrupt a good sleep routine. If we can understand more about the day-night rhythm of our brain, we can train it to sleep better. Yes, sleep is yet another learned behavior that we must learn to do well to feel good.

Understanding Sleep

Circadian rhythms are natural body rhythms over a twenty-four-hour period that tell your body when to sleep and when to be awake. This "master clock" is made of approximately twenty thousand brain cells in the suprachiasmatic nucleus inside the hypothalamus, close to where the optic nerves from the eyes cross. These rhythms—with the help of the hypothalamus—regulate other biological patterns, such as body temperature and hormone patterns, hunger and thirst, fatigue, and, of course, sleep. You can see how if one rhythm is disrupted, it easily affects the others. Stressful events and late-night eating can trigger hormones to release in a different pattern, keeping you awake at night and tired during the day. Our bodies do best with regular routines of sleeping and waking, eating and digesting, and moving and resting.

How well do you sleep?

Do you:

- ⮑ Fall asleep within twenty to thirty minutes?
- ⮑ Wake fewer than four times per night?
- ⮑ Wake up without an alarm clock?
- ⮑ Wake at the same time every day?
- ⮑ Wake up feeling rested?
- ⮑ Sleep for at least ten hours per day for children, eight for teens?

Stages of Sleep

Regular, restorative sleep means getting Delta wave (deep) sleep each night.

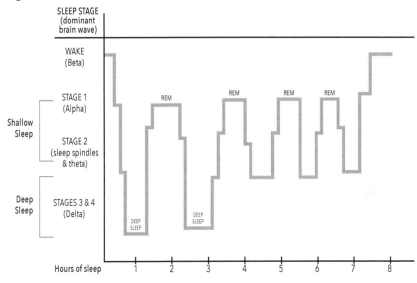

One of the most important things you can do to have a lifetime of mostly good sleep is to keep a regular routine, which translates into rarely sleeping in on weekends or taking humongous midday naps. I know, this is a tough sell, especially with teenagers, who may believe that if you don't get that Saturday morning slumber until noon, you will never "catch up." But those delicious habits are part of the reason you are not getting restful sleep during the rest of the week. "Catching up" on sleep can contribute to the problem of insomnia. Understanding the different stages of sleep architecture will help you understand why you need to keep a general routine—even if it sounds absurd, un-American, or inhumane.

Most people have heard of rapid eye movement, or REM, sleep, and although it is important, it is not deep sleep. There are five categories of brain waves (measured in Hz) that characterize our sleep and waking states:

- Beta waves (the most rapid type) allow you to do things such as focus enough to comprehend this sentence.
- Alpha waves are slower and reflect more of a relaxed awake state.

- Theta waves are next, a bit slower still, and are predominant in the beginning of deeper sleep.

- Delta waves are the slowest and dominate during deep sleep.

- REM sleep usually happens in shallow stages of sleep and helps us encode information from the day into our memory banks to be useful information we can retrieve tomorrow (provided we have a good night sleep).

Alpha and beta waves are present in shallow stages of sleep. Theta waves come when you are deeply relaxed and possibly moving toward delta sleep. Delta wave sleep, or deep sleep, is why we feel rested when we do sleep well. Human growth hormone is released during this stage—necessary for cell reproduction and regeneration—and when our best healing takes place. It is possible to sleep all night long but wake up feeling terrible. This is usually because of too much shallow sleep (stage one, two, and REM) and not enough deep (delta) sleep. We cycle through these stages again and again throughout the night, from shallow to deep to REM to shallow to deep to REM and so on—about every ninety minutes or so. Contrary to popular belief, most people do not need more REM sleep. IBSers have twice as much REM sleep as people without IBS—displaying more sympathetic nervous system activity (stress response). They may benefit from training their brains to get more deep, delta-wave sleep.

How to Get Better Quality Sleep

1) **Keep a routine:** If you go to bed early or sleep in, your body will naturally calculate that it has had enough deep sleep and stay in shallow sleep, possibly dipping into deep sleep just as you need to be up and at 'em. The same thing happens if you nap too late or too much during the day. Pick a wake-up time to keep every day of the week. Even if you stay out one night and miss your usual bedtime, wake up at the same time the next morning. You may be tired that day—but by not sleeping in, you will avoid disrupting your circadian rhythm and have better sleep the following nights.

2) **No dozing on the couch:** this too can throw off the rhythm. Your

brain calculates it just had a power nap, then you crawl into bed and cannot fall asleep.

3) **Get out of bed if you are not sleeping:** use classical conditioning (pair bed and sleep together) to train your brain to sleep when your head hits the pillow. As comfy and cozy as your bed may be, it is not the place for doing anything other than sleeping. (You don't sit on the toilet if you don't plan to use it, right?)

4) **Worry somewhere else:** Being given the chance to talk about worries and fears earlier in the day may make your child's fears less intense at nighttime. Worrying about not sleeping can be another worry to add to the list. Some people need to get up out of bed and worry somewhere else for fifteen minutes or so before they try to lie down and sleep again. When you become sleepy, go back to bed. Then, if you are not asleep in twenty to thirty minutes, get up out of bed again and read until you are tired.

5) **Exercise:** On days you get cardiovascular exercise (get that heart rate up while moving rhythmically), you get more delta sleep. If you are not physically active enough during the day, your brain, although tired, may not have a strong enough signal to knock you into deep sleep for very long.

6) **Diet:** There is some evidence that eating fewer simple carbohydrates (processed foods) at dinner will allow for more delta wave sleep. (High simple carbohydrate diets are associated with many other health problems, too.) If you are not already, especially avoid sugary, fatty, and high carbohydrate foods at nighttime. Why give your guts anything else to worry about at nighttime? Your digestive tract needs sleep too.

7) **Be aware of certain medications and alcohol:** Narcotic pain medications and long-term use of benzodiazapines can zap deep sleep, leaving you with poor sleep with or without the medications. Steroids, allergy medications, alcohol, and anything with caffeine can keep you from sleeping and sleeping deeply.

chapter 9

Children between the ages of five and ten years old need approximately ten to eleven hours of sleep per night, while teens need a little bit less. Getting enough sleep is important; however, getting good quality sleep is even more important. Although our circadian rhythms are naturally encoded in our genetic code, cues may be necessary to retrain our brains to get restful sleep at nighttime and feel alert during the daytime.

A good sleep environment must be:

- **Safe:** Feeling safe is a must or the body does not receive the signal that it is OK to sleep. You can't be anxious and feel safe at the same time.

- **Dark:** Darkness at night helps to signal to the body through hormone shifts that it is time to sleep. Help the wake-up hormones by getting ten to fifteen minutes of real sunlight each morning sitting near a window or going outside.

- **Quiet:** If noise bothers you, invest in earplugs or use white noise, such as a fan, to block out intermittent noises that pull an anxious brain out of deep sleep.

- **Solely for sleep:** The bed is not for homework, reading, television, thinking, or playtime. Keep your bed for sleep only. Do other activities somewhere else.

- **Routine:** Avoid sleeping in late, as this disrupts your body's natural sleep cycles. If you must stay up late once in a while, still wake at your normal time the next morning to restart the routine and avoid "catching up."

- **Caffeine free:** Avoid caffeine, soda, chocolate or other stimulants, especially after noon (especially sodas and energy drinks).

- **Relaxing:** Create a relaxing bedtime routine. This may include reading a book, listening to calming music, brushing teeth, or bathing. Do the same routine each night, starting at the same time, allowing plenty of time to settle down from the busy day. (You may know someone who switches off like a light switch at night, but many children need cues to help prepare them for sleep.)

- **Screen free:** Avoid televisions, computers, or other bright lights one to two hours before bed. Light stimulates the brain chemicals into thinking it is time to be awake.

Once you have established a routine, your child should be able to wake up naturally without an alarm clock. If your child has trouble falling asleep, use one of the relaxation techniques from chapter 5 for ten to fifteen minutes each night.

What is your sleep score?

You can calculate your sleep efficiency by subtracting how many hours of sleep you actually get from the amount of time you spend in bed attempting to sleep.

Example: Bedtime 9 p.m., wake 7 a.m., asleep seven hours. Sleep efficiency = 7/10, which is 70 percent of the time you are asleep in bed. One way to improve sleep efficiency is to spend less time in bed. If you go to bed at 9 p.m. but are not falling asleep for the first hour, do not go to bed until 10 p.m. Once you are falling asleep more quickly on a regular basis, you can start going to bed earlier.

CHAPTER SUMMARY

- Your child, depending on his age and activity level, needs approximately eight to twelve hours of sleep. A regular sleep schedule is best, for example, bedtime around 9 p.m., waking about 7 a.m.

- Circadian rhythms are natural body rhythms over a twenty-four-hour period that tell your body when to sleep and when to be awake. This is the "master clock" of the sleep-wake rhythm.

- Avoid long naps, especially late in the day.

- Do not stay in bed if you are not sleepy. Lying awake will only make you more anxious and annoyed. Dozing in and out is not good sleep and is worse than just getting up and going back to bed when sleepy.

- Avoid sleeping in on the weekends.

chapter 9

- Get plenty of exercise during the daytime.

- Certain medications and alcohol can decrease good quality deep sleep.

- A relaxing bedtime routine is very important for training your brain to sleep when you want it to.

- Use a worry place somewhere other than bed to get the worries worked out.

- The best sleep environment is safe, dark, quiet, solely for sleep, routine, caffeine free, relaxing, and screen free.

❓ QUESTIONS FOR YOUR FAMILY

Each family member can take a turn answering the following questions.

1) What will you change in your bedtime routine to make it more peaceful?

2) What hours work best for you to go to bed and wake up seven days per week?

CHAPTER 10

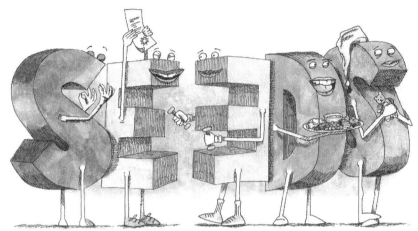

Socializing and Planting the SEEDS for Success

Behavior Change and Goal Setting

We have talked about many ways to improve your young one's life with IBS. Many self-management techniques for IBS are similar to other healthy behaviors we all may try to maintain throughout a life span. It has not escaped us that changing bad habits to healthy ones can be difficult. But don't make it harder than it is; when it is challenging, accept that and move forward. It will get easier.

How easy is it to add regular relaxation, assertive communication, exercise, a healthy diet and routine sleep to your daily life? It's not! Healthy habits are difficult for most people to incorporate into a daily routine, not to mention all the other things we might be trying to do in life: learn to play a musical instrument, be nicer, sing better, stand taller, grow a garden, write a book, climb a mountain, finish school, or save money. On the other hand, obsessing about doing everything "right" will not help either.

The keys to making and maintaining healthy habits are:

- Specific goals
- Small changes over time
- Frequent rewards
- Positive self-talk
- Information
- Evaluating what works
- Problem solving what does not work
- Persistence (try and try again)
- Social support
- Making it fun

Making specific goals is important because specificity guides us on how to go about meeting each goal. Think about the management of symptoms such as diarrhea, constipation, and bloating. A goal of having fewer tummy aches or less diarrhea is too general and may not be realistic unless other changes are already in place. A goal of practicing diaphragmatic breathing for ten minutes per day at 7 a.m. and 7 p.m. is specific and much more realistic since it is something within personal control.

Realistic expectations are also important. Small changes are more realistic than a New Year's resolution type of goal. Light bulb moments make great television, but more often, people change little by little, after several attempts. The average smoker quits three times before he stays quit. Huge changes tend to be short lived and then viewed as failures. We naturally revert back to familiar habits after feeling the discouragement of several failed attempts and are left with less motivation to try again. Instead, we could learn from setbacks and remind our children, it's OK to "fail." You don't need to protect them from feeling the letdown of failure, but they do need to learn how to do their best, handle failures, and move forward.

Motivation is one of the best predictors of behavior change. Rewards are important to keep us motivated along the way to creating good habits. Planning fun activities each day can be used as rewards. Fun social activities also keep your child involved, which dramatically reduces the likelihood of chronic anxiety and depression. Help your child develop a hobby or interest and link it to a reward that does not sabotage the efforts toward his or her goal. For example, snack food as a reward is typically not a good idea as it can worsen IBS; however, a new Wii dance game could be a reward itself for movement.

Be aware of how rewarding illness behavior is different from being supportive. Parents sometimes inadvertently increase their child's pain by giving him or her positive reinforcement for illness behaviors out of pity or guilt. (Example: giving in to more television when your daughter has a tummy ache versus emotional support and encouragement to rest and then tackle homework.) Children will naturally learn to do what they are rewarded for doing, whether or not you are rewarding them intentionally. Sometimes you may feel frustrated as a parent and withdraw emotional support. Although this is unintentional, it may lead to more displays of sick behavior in order to get parental attention. The type of attention and limit setting make all the difference.

Observing your self-talk and that of your child is also important, especially when trying something new. Setbacks and flare-ups are normal, but all-or-nothing thinking can lead to frustration at the first sign of failure, thwarting any future attempts. Remind each other that this is a process, and although you cannot change the past, together you can change what you do right now. Help your child track small signs of progress, normalize setbacks, and give lots of encouragement to continue.

If you feel stuck in a rut of bad habits (we all have some), do not hesitate to ask others for advice and seek out the best information available. This could be from books, the Internet, or people. It might be a neighbor, friend, family member, rabbi, pastor, or health care worker. Be open to other people's suggestions—with the awareness that the information they share is not necessarily true—and decide for yourself what you want to try. Partner with your child and try a variety of ideas to find out what works for your family. When something does not work right away, problem-solve, make changes as needed, and try, try, again. Understanding and compassion for each other are key.

Socializing and Fun

One antidote to stress is having fun and feeling increasingly connected to family, friends, school, community, and the larger society. This point was brought home to us when Steven, a twelve-year-old boy in our program, said, "I don't feel like I'm a freak anymore." Before SEEDS he felt isolated, different, and disconnected from others because of his IBS. Children with IBS and its potentially embarrassing symptoms internalize the stress around them and start believing they have done something wrong or are bad people, or they wouldn't have these problems. They must be reassured through words and actions that this is not true. Helping children build a sense of connectedness with others protects them from the pitfalls of the world—whether reducing depression and isolation or preventing reckless or illegal behaviors.

Compassion and empathy will build over time as they learn from you what really matters. Being able to reach out to others will help them build confidence, just as learning to take good care of their own needs will help them be able to reach out to others. Having fun with others teaches them to celebrate together and that they do not have to suffer alone. Some ideas for increasing social connections and community include:

- Volunteer opportunities
- Homeless feeding programs
- Church fellowship events
- Community centers
- Clubs and camps
- Family field trips
- Day trips with friends
- Playing outdoors
- Playing or listening to music

Building connections can increase our compassion for others and ourselves and predicts better physical and psychological health. Research shows people who feel emotional support from others contract fewer colds, recover faster after a heart attack, and experience less pain and depression. The number of friends one has does not necessarily predict better health, but rather the perceived closeness of supportive relationships. Generally, it is quality over quantity as long as there is more than one person you can lean on.

Children are underestimated for their contribution to the world. Some adult guidance and enthusiasm can go a long way. Children have started charities, invented ingenious machines, and have demonstrated amazing acts of kindness. In your family, better social connectivity may mean volunteering with your children to help others or regularly visiting the elderly neighbor. GPAs of 4.0 may predict who gets into college, but not who does well in the workforce. Getting along with others allows us to feel joy at home, school, and work, reducing depression, anxiety, and the physical manifestations of stress.

The Internet, computer games, Wii, television, and iPhones™ are all tools, and, as with any tool, it depends how we use these things in our lives that determines whether they improve our health or lead to more problems. Technology can help us stay connected with friends or provide entertainment and enjoyment, but it is easy and tempting to overuse technology in lieu of things that bring us lasting pleasure. We need daily activities that move our bodies and stimulate our brains. Isolation or anxious hovering contributes to more abdominal discomfort by allowing children to focus on feeling ill rather than on the good things life has to offer.

One of the necessities to successfully manage IBS is for children to have fun—a lot of it. This does not at all mean foregoing all structure and discipline. It simply means that with appropriate guidelines of common sense and safety, almost anything can be enjoyable. Children (and adults) need a lot of fun. So whether it is beginning an exercise program, changing dinner menus, or just hanging out with the family—fun needs to be part of it. The experience of pleasure releases endorphins, the body's natural painkillers, and fun allows neuroplasticity to take place to our advantage!

chapter 10

Making healthy behaviors into habits is easier with support from other people. Here are a few ways to increase social connections that help us make and keep healthy changes:

- Find (or be) a friend or family member who will play with your child for a daily dose of movement.

- Eat together as a family. This makes it quality time together while engaging in healthy behaviors.

- Host a family game night on a regular basis.

- Get involved with something you care about in your community—such as a community garden.

- Be a role model. Remember, children will learn much more by what you do than by what you say.

Over the next few months, Sara came to realize that her sensitive gut felt much better when her life was in balance: not overscheduled, yet engaged in many fun activities; not pushing herself to overachieve, but staying active on a regular basis; eating regular meals and limiting trigger foods, such as simple sugars and fatty foods; resting when she felt overwhelmed and keeping a regular sleep schedule. She was able to talk with her best friend when she was having a flare-up, and they watched their favorite comedy movie together.

After learning about her body's brain-gut connection, Sara appreciates the big job her brain-gut system has to do daily and now accepts that flare-ups come and go. She prepares herself ahead of time when school starts or ends, taking her time to readjust to the changes. When an unexpected stress leaps her way, she keeps her regular sleep and exercise routine, adds in more relaxation, and works on keeping close social ties to her family and friends for support. When she feels misunderstood, she speaks up. She reminds herself that flare-ups are temporary and not her fault. With these skills, she is able to attend school most days, even with some tummy pain and diarrhea. She does her best to be aware of the things that trigger anxiety and cope with them better. Sara is reassured and more confident about managing her life with IBS, and IBS no longer controls her.

CHAPTER SUMMARY

- Changes last longer when we have support, when goals are specific, when rewards are used, when we have accurate information, and when we persist despite setbacks.

- Research shows us again and again that to maximize our health, we need to feel connected socially.

- Make it a priority to spend time with family, friends, and community, and to participate in activities that you and your child care about.

- Having fun increases endorphins, the body's natural painkillers, and we feel less pain. Helping others reduces pain and improves mood.

? QUESTIONS FOR YOUR FAMILY

Each family member can take a turn answering the following questions.

1) When will we take time each week to have fun as a family?

2) What activities will we do together?

3) Who are you other than a person who has IBS?

chapter 10

Frequently Asked Questions about Functional Gastrointestinal Disorders

1. Is IBS a psychological or a physical problem?

Yes. Both. Over time, psychological or emotional stress can change the way the brain processes signals from the digestive tract, resulting in heightened awareness of discomfort, called visceral hypersensitivity.

2. What is the cause of IBS?

IBS symptoms are the result of visceral (inside organ) hypersensitivity and a decreased capacity of the digestive tract to accommodate food and gas.

3. Who gets IBS?

School-aged children and adults; 80 percent of them are female.

4. Should we keep going to see the doctor for IBS?

No, but do listen to what your doctor has to say. The more unnecessary doctor visits, the higher likelihood of having unnecessary procedures and surgeries that can lead to other problems. (And, yes, as doctors, we are trying to put ourselves out of business.)

5. Could the symptoms be from a food allergy?

This occurs less than 5 percent of the time and is usually very obvious to a pediatrician who has taken a medical history and learned about the child's reaction.

6. Should we track all the foods we eat to see what is causing the IBS?

Being aware of what you are putting into your body is a good thing. However, tracking every food and every symptom can lead children to be obsessed with identifying food as the culprit, which, besides sugary and fatty foods, it usually is not. You can help your child eat according to her symptoms and eat a healthy diet overall without becoming consumed by food.

7. Breakfast is the most important meal of the day, so why is it so hard to eat?

The gut may not be ready, and poor sleep patterns leave the stomach very sensitive. Introduce small amounts of easy-to-digest foods. See chapter 8 for details.

8. The food issue is so confusing, so what should we avoid and what should we eat?

The best research shows that avoiding too much fructose will help, especially high fructose corn syrup in processed foods.

9. Should my child take probiotics?

There is some evidence that it helps with bloating.

10. Will my child always have IBS?

IBS is a chronic condition, and about 75 percent of sufferers continue to have symptoms on and off throughout their lives; however, we now know how to minimize their impact.

11. Should my child stay home from school because of stomach pain or other IBS symptoms?

Generally speaking, no. Every child has different needs, but overall, IBS and anxiety become worse the more school is missed.

12. How do you know it isn't cancer or something else more horrible?

Bad things tend to surface early and show up on lab tests. It is rare to find out later that symptoms are something other than IBS, once IBS is diagnosed. Some parents become obsessed with finding the "something else," resulting in more frustration, anxiety, depression, unnecessary procedures, and incidental findings.

13. Should my child be exercising?

Movement is essential. Endorphins from exercise help reduce stress, improve sleep, and block pain pathways. Playing is the best exercise for children without the pressure of a regimented "workout."

14. OK, I know what we should be doing, but how do I get my child to do these things?

Set up your environment to support a regular routine of eating, sleeping, exercise, socializing, and relaxation. Since children copy their parents' health care behaviors, be a good role model of health. If something needs changing, make gradual and realistic goals that have the natural reward of feeling better long term.

15. I think I get it, but my spouse and I are not on the same page. What do we do?

The marked improvement in IBS symptoms will support the diagnosis and path you should take. If you disagree, discuss it away from your children and find common ground. If there is a lot of conflict in your home, seek professional help, as it is likely adding stress to your child's existing fears.

16. What else can I do as a parent of a child with IBS?

Be supportive and confident, be a good role model, and listen to what your child has to say.

Glossary

Anterior cingulate cortex: Part of the brain that helps us detect problems. It also regulates emotions and blood pressure.

Biopsychosocial model: A scientific model first developed by Dr. George Engel that systematically considers biological, psychological (thoughts, emotions, behaviors), and social factors and their complex interactions in understanding health and illness.

Brain-gut axis: Relationship between the brain and intestines, best understood by the biopsychosocial model.

Chyme: Semidigested food that is being passed out of the small intestine.

Digestive enzymes: Substances that help break down large molecules (usually food) into smaller molecules.

Disimpaction: Removing fecal matter (poop) that has not been eliminated naturally, sometimes manually or with enemas.

Dorsal horns: Part of the spinal column associated with sensory neurons (versus motor neurons).

Duodenum: The first portion of the small intestine.

Endorphins: Chemicals produced by the brain that reduce the perception of pain; the body's natural painkillers. Also called endogenous opioids.

Enmeshed: Entangled, overly connected in relationship to someone else, not separate.

Heart rate variability: The beat-to-beat change in heart rate, reflecting adaptability and health of the nervous system.

Intestinal motility: Ability to move chyme, stool and gas spontaneously while consuming energy.

Large bowel or large intestines: Organ that absorbs water from remaining indigestible food and passes the rest out as waste.

Macronutrients: Nutrients in diet that are required in large amounts, such as protein, fat, carbohydrates, and macrominerals, such as calcium, potassium, and magnesium.

Neuroplasticity: The capacity of the nervous system to regenerate or make new neuronal connections (nerve connections).

Pain gate: The chemical pathway by which our body sends our brain messages about pain.

Serotonin: A chemical in the brain and gut derived from tryptophan that is used for memory, sleep, mood, and other neurological processes.

Small bowel or small intestines: The narrow, longer part of the intestines, comprising of the duodenum, jejunum, and ileum that serves to digest food and absorb nutrients.

Visceral hypersensitivity: Visceral refers to internal organs, and hypersensitivity refers to information flooding the brain with pain sensations that are stronger than expected.

Index

Further Reading

BOOKS

Boundaries: When to Say Yes, How to Say No to Take Control of Your Life, by Henry Cloud and John Townsend (Zondervan, 2002).

Conquering Irritable Bowel Syndrome: A guide to liberating those suffering with chronic stomach or bowel problems, by Nicholas J. Talley.

Everyday Blessings: The Inner Work of Mindful Parenting, by Kabat-Zinn, M. & Kabat-Zinn, J. (1998).

Master Your IBS: An 8-week plan to control the symptoms of irritable bowel syndrome, by Pamela Barney, AGA Press.

The Mindful Way Through Depression: Freeing Yourself from Chronic Unhappiness, by M. Williams, J. Teasedale, Z. Segal, and J. Kabat-Zinn (2007).

Parenting with Love and Logic, by Foster Cline and Jim Fay (NavPress, 2006).

The Relaxation and Stress Reduction Workbook, by Davis, M., Eschelman, E. & McKay, M. (2002).

The Trigger Point Therapy Workbook, by C. Davies (2004).

INTERNET RESOURCES

The Feeding and Eating Experts: www.ellynsatter.com

Family Support: www.makinghealthyfamilies.com

International Foundation for Functional Gastrointestinal Disorders: www.iffgd.org

JOURNAL ARTICLES

Talley, N.J. (2012). Dietary Mondification as a Treatment for Irritable Bowel Syndrome. Advances in Nutrition, 8(8), 552-554.

Eswaran, S., Goel, A., Chey, W.D. (2013). What Role Does Wheat Play in the Symptoms of Irritable Bowel Syndrome? Gastroenterology & Hepatology, 9 (2), 85-92.

American College of Gastroenterology Task Force on IBS (2009). An Evidence-

Based Systematic Review on the Management of Irritable Bowel Syndrome. Supplement to the American Journal of Gastroenterology, 104 (1).

Kaptchuk, T.J., Friedlander, E., Kelley, J.M., Sanchez, M.N., Kokkotou, E., Singer, J.P., Kowalczykowski, M., Miller, F.G., Kirsch, I., Lembo, A.J., (2010). Placebos without Deception: A Randomized Controlled Trial in Irritable Bowel Syndrome. PLoS ONE, 5(12), 1-7.

Wu, J. (2010). *Complementary and Alternative Medicine for the Treatment of Irritable Bowel Syndrome: Facts or Myths? Gastroenterology & Hepatology,* 6 (11), 705-711.

Jarrett, M.E., Burr, R.L., Cain, K.C., Rothermel, J.D., Landis, C.A., Heitkemper, M.M., (2008). *Autonomic Nervous System Function During Sleep Among Women with Irritable Bowel Syndrome. Digestive Disease Sciences,* 53, 694-703.

Palsson, O.S., Whitehead, W.E., (2012). *Psychological Treatments in Functional Gastrointestinal Disorders: A primer for the Gastroenterologist. Clinical Gastroenterology and Hepatology,* 11(2), 208-216.

Thomas, J.R., Nanda, R., Shu, L.H. (2012). *A FODMAP Diet Update: Craze or Credible? Practical Gastroenterology,* 37-46.

further
reading

36347307R00082

Made in the USA
San Bernardino, CA
20 May 2019